ONCE A
GIANT

ONCE A
GIANT

A Story of Victory, Tragedy,
and Life After Football

GARY MYERS

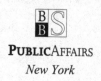

PublicAffairs
New York

PublicAffairs
Hachette Book Group
1290 Avenue of the Americas, New York, NY 10104
www.publicaffairsbooks.com
@Public_Affairs

Printed in the United States of America
First Edition: September 2023
First Trade Paperback Edition: November 2024
Published by PublicAffairs, an imprint of Hachette Book Group, Inc. The PublicAffairs name and logo is a registered trademark of the Hachette Book Group.

The Hachette Speakers Bureau provides a wide range of authors for speaking events. To find out more, go to hachettespeakersbureau.com or email HachetteSpeakers@hbgusa.com.

PublicAffairs books may be purchased in bulk for business, educational, or promotional use. For more information, please contact your local bookseller or the Hachette Book Group Special Markets Department at special.markets@hbgusa.com.

The publisher is not responsible for websites (or their content) that are not owned by the publisher.

Print book interior design by Jeff Williams.

Library of Congress Cataloging-in-Publication Data
Names: Myers, Gary, 1954 July 1– author.
Title: Once a Giant : a story of victory, tragedy, and life after football / Gary Myers.
Description: First edition. | New York, N.Y. : PublicAffairs, 2023.
Identifiers: LCCN 2022060911 | ISBN 9781541702394 (hardcover) | ISBN 9781541702417 (ebook)
Subjects: LCSH: New York Giants (Football team)—History. | Super Bowl (21st : 1987 : Pasadena, Calif.) | Football players—United States—Conduct of life. | Football players—United States—Retirement. | Football injuries. | Football players—United States—Biography. | Football coaches—United States—Biography.
Classification: LCC GV956.N4 M94 2023 | DDC 796.332/64097471—dc23/eng/20221222
LC record available at https://lccn.loc.gov/2022060911

ISBNs: 9781541702394 (hardcover), 9781541702417 (ebook), 9781541702400 (paperback)

LSC-C

Printing 1, 2024

To Allison, Michelle, Emily, and Andrew

CONTENTS

Photographs follow page 120.

ONCE A
GIANT

INTRODUCTION

Parcells Savings and Loan

Bill Parcells has a paternal pride that is all over his face as he gives a tour of his office right off the garage of his winter home in Tequesta in Palm Beach County. It serves as a museum with artifacts of his coaching life: two Super Bowl championships with the New York Giants, a Super Bowl appearance with the New England Patriots, and playoff games with the New York Jets and Dallas Cowboys.

The story of the brotherhood of the beloved and iconic 1986 Super Bowl champion New York Football Giants is dramatically told by the pictures on the walls. Safety Kenny Hill was the only member of the team (coach included) who had previously been part of a Super Bowl championship, so they would learn how to depend on one another to win from Parcells, a master motivator and lifelong Giants fan from New Jersey who grew up down the street from Giants Stadium in Hasbrouck Heights and Oradell.

Parcells has a colorful story for each photograph of his former players, his "guys." You can sense his affection as he rattles off their names.

"The great Phil Simms"—the quarterback who pitched a nearly perfect game with his twenty-two-of-twenty-five performance in Super Bowl XXI on January 25, 1987.

"Lawrence Taylor. I love that guy"—the best, and most troubled, player he coached.

"Jim Burt. Now that's a character"—the wiseass with whom he traded one-liners.

"Mark Bavaro. Great kid. Tough. Love him"—the tight end who returned in the same game against the Saints in 1986 after he broke his jaw.

"Banksie"—Carl Banks, a phenomenal linebacker on two Giants championship teams.

Parcells is the only coach in NFL history to take four different teams to the postseason. Of course, not many coaches are afforded the opportunity to coach four different teams. They don't get fired three times and then have billionaire owners step up and figure, why not, maybe he'll get it right the fourth time. Parcells's journey was highly unusual. He turned around four programs and always departed on his own terms, a rarity in the coaching profession, leaving players and fans wanting more. He did once come dangerously close to being fired by general manager George Young after he was 3–12–1 in his first season as an NFL head coach with the Giants in 1983. It was no oversight that Young was omitted from Parcells's long and winding Pro Football Hall of Fame induction speech in 2013. It was petty and pointless, considering Young had been dead for more than a decade.

Parcells's winter retirement home in Florida is immaculate, even more impressive since he's in his early eighties, divorced, and lives alone. There's a deck in the back separated from the Intercoastal by trees and shrubs, providing a nice view for unwinding after his early morning workout at the gym and frequent rounds of golf. His home is around the corner from Bagel Bistro, a nondescript eatery in a strip mall on US-1, which serves as his favorite meeting spot with Bill Belichick, the defensive coordinator on his Super Bowl teams with the Giants, who is coming to town in a few days.

"Bill loves that place. We're getting together Saturday morning at 6:30," Parcells said. "He usually has something he wants to discuss with me."

Big Bill and Little Bill look like typical Florida retirees getting together for bagels and lox early in the morning, except that Belichick, in his early seventies, is still coaching the Patriots. An early-bird football fan who walks in and hears these legends talking ball would do a double take. They long ago made their peace after a falling out when Belichick left the Jets in 2000 instead of succeeding Parcells as coach, as his contract stipulated. Little Bill worked his way to New England, the reverse of what Big Bill had done, having walked away from the Patriots to take the Jets' head coaching job in 1997. Parcells is now a valuable sounding board for Belichick, just as he is for the long list of coaches who consult with him on issues ranging from handling unexpected problems on their team to career advice.

Parcells even recommended Belichick move into the Jupiter Yacht Club condo development, where Parcells had a winter home at the time. Belichick followed his advice, once inadvertently flooding his former boss's apartment when a water pipe burst in Belichick's sixth-floor unit two floors above Parcells. Belichick was not home and maintenance came to the rescue.

Parcells's hobby is owning thoroughbred racehorses, and the wall outside his office is lined with pictures of his ponies. He also has a home in Saratoga in upstate New York, not far from the famed Saratoga Race Course, where he can be found most summer afternoons watching the horses run. When possible, he tries to name his horses after his former players. It's one way to hold onto his Giants years, which mean so much to him. Mark Bavaro and Maurice Carthon have been so honored. And he named one of his horses Tuggle, after running back John Tuggle, the very last player picked in the 1983 draft. Tuggle died of blood vessel cancer at the age of twenty-five on the eve of the 1986 Super Bowl season but lives on in Parcells's memories. Parcells also had a horse named Once A Giant that he sold in a claims race in 2022.

"When are you going to name one after me?" someone shouted from the back of the room at a Parcells speaking engagement in New York in 2016.

At first, Parcells was confused about who was giving him a hard time. The lights were off except for those on the stage, and the heckler was ducking behind the guests in the last row of the theater. Parcells eventually saw it was Banks and laughed. He later explained another horse owner beat him to the Banks name. Not so with Simms.

"I have a two-year-old named Golden Simms," he said. "I called Simms and told him, 'That horse better run faster than you!'"

When Parcells informed his quarterback he now had a namesake with four legs, Simms asked whether the thoroughbred's name was Horse's Ass.

Football was fun for the '86 Giants. They were bonded for life by the Lombardi Trophy and their diamond championship rings.

They care about one another. They take care of one another. There is a built-in support system among the teammates. Text chains, card shows, reunions, they talk and see each other frequently. They take each other to doctor's appointments. Wives who were not part of the team in 1986 are amazed, witnessing a side of their husbands they've never seen when they are around their teammates at reunions: hugging, joking, acting like kids. At the twenty-fifth reunion, Parcells said running back Lee Rouson's wife, Lisa, came up to him.

"Mr. Parcells, can I ask you a question?" she said.

"Sure," he said.

They were standing off to the side in a private room at halftime on reunion weekend.

"What is this?" she said, looking at her husband and teammates acting like they were twenty-five years old again.

"You know, that's a very good question," he said.

He paused for a moment.

"This is a group of people who are bonded together, that have accomplished something together and that's their guys. And they're going to always be their guys. And it's a lifelong thing. And it's never going to change and that's really the way it is. It's not going to change," Parcells said.

Nobody in the room would disagree.

"It's wonderful to have extended family like that," said co-captain George Martin, who was a father figure to many players, old and young.

A few years later, Rouson's wife called Parcells and requested he record a video birthday greeting on his cell phone for Lee. He was delighted she asked. If a player in 1986 was setting the odds on Parcells ever recording birthday greetings on his phone—or even knowing how to do it—they would have been longer than the odds of Golden Simms winning the Kentucky Derby.

"You can't buy into this fraternity," Burt said.

Football has given them so much. Football has taken so much away.

Life after football has been cruel to far too many of them. The transition and adjustment to the next phase of life can be overwhelming. Achieving the ultimate victory of winning a Super Bowl and being among a group of guys who truly love one another is hard to replicate, and it creates an emptiness almost no matter what comes next. Emotionally, intellectually, physically, and financially it can be the highlight of their lives. Bavaro admits he's never found anything else that he's good at after he retired. It creates a difficult transition filled with all the dangerous ramifications of a career in a violent sport.

Suicidal thoughts. Death. Bodies breaking down. Mental health disorders. Money problems.

═══

THE NFL CITES a study that projects the average life expectancy of an NFL player to be 77.5 years and the average for men in the general population to be 74.7 years. That number does not account for quality of life, however. Another study shows that players who would be categorized as obese—generally offensive and defensive linemen—are dying faster than their teammates. And another says the life expectancy of professional football players is the mid- to late fifties, about twenty years fewer than the average population.

This is not a problem unique to the 1986 Giants. It threatens and scares football players of yesterday, today, and tomorrow. What does life look like in their fifties and sixties and seventies? Will they be able to walk? Will they be afflicted with early dementia? Will they be haunted by suicidal thoughts? Will they have any money?

That's the stage of life for the '86 Giants as it now approaches four decades since they partied in Pasadena. They are growing old together. There was no handbook when they retired with directions on how to find their way to the next phase of their life. Their NFL health insurance covered most of them for only one year after retirement. The first question at reunions used to be checking up on each other's kids. Then as the years passed, it moved to grandchildren. Now they ask about doctor's appointments and referrals and scheduled surgeries. "Amazing how it's changed," center Bart Oates said. For every player whose bones make weird noises as he crawls out of bed in the morning, there are teammates worrying about CTE, chronic traumatic encephalopathy, a degenerative brain disease that can't be officially diagnosed until after death. CTE has been linked to traumatic brain injury caused by concussions, resulting in depression and desperation that led to suicide for former players Junior Seau, Dave Duerson, Andre Waters, and Greg Clark, among others.

Bobby Johnson, a wide receiver who is a recovering crack addict, was asked which of his Giants teammates are worried about the brain disorder. "All of us," he said. "It ain't just from the NFL. It's from college and high school all the way down to Pee Wee." The dangers of head trauma hit home for Bavaro, the Giants indestructible tight end: His wife, Susan, an attorney, believes the Covid virus attacked his brain, which was compromised by Bavaro's numerous concussions during his football career. The impact of Covid was debilitating. Dark thoughts overwhelmed him. Bavaro was teammates with Duerson at Notre Dame and later with the Giants, and Waters was a teammate in his last NFL stop in Philadelphia. Duerson and Waters killed themselves: Duerson with a gunshot to the chest, Waters with a gunshot to the head. Their brains were donated for scientific and medical research and subsequently diagnosed with CTE.

Leonard Marshall, one of the defensive enforcers on the '86 Giants, is convinced he has CTE and says he's been diagnosed with early-stage Parkinson's disease. He was among the more than five thousand retired players listed in the settlement of the $1 billion concussion lawsuit brought against the NFL that was finalized on January 7, 2017. The maximum payout per player is $5 million, but Marshall has not yet been notified what he will be awarded. Oates, the leader of the "Suburbanites," the all-white starting offensive line, and now the president of the NFL Alumni Association, believes 30–40 percent of his former teammates exhibit traits of Parkinson's—rigidity, balance issues, slight tremors, shrinking handwriting, gait problems. After much internal turmoil, Marshall has elected to donate his brain for CTE research after he passes. "The game is what it is," Hall of Fame linebacker Harry Carson said. "It is a collision sport. When you have bodies flying around at high rates of speed, bad things are going to happen."

Carson, who has fought his way through post-concussion syndrome, spoke to Congress about traumatic brain injuries and petitioned the surgeon general for a warning on children's permission slips that football can be dangerous to their neurological health. He wants to ensure parents are aware of potential issues that could occur twenty or thirty years down the road.

Nobody, of course, forced these men to play football at any level and subject themselves to the dangers of the game. Only the fortunate few are skilled enough to make it to the NFL. They signed up to play in the league in the '80s knowing the risk of tearing the anterior cruciate ligament in their knees or needing multiple back surgeries or ripping up their shoulders. Injuring their brain was not part of the conversation. Teams weren't avoiding educating their players about the long-term danger of head trauma as much as they were just as ill informed as the players.

"We boys think it's a game. We men know it's a game played for money," Marshall said. "Cognitive impairment, traumatic brain injury, CTE, Alzheimer's, early-stage Parkinson's, any of that stuff, those words were never uttered in association with the game." In our conversation, Marshall was frustrated trying to recall what year he broke his wrist. Finally, he narrowed it down to 1987 or 1988. "I can't remember because of my brain," he said.

It's impossible to walk away from the game mentally or physically unscathed. If the '86 Giants had foresight, they saved money, but with salaries just a fraction of what they are today, they needed to find a job after football, preferably one that provided health insurance. Ask Marshall which body part hurts and the conversation is lengthy. "Shit bothers me," he said. "What am I going to do about it? Complain and cry in my beer?" Marshall survived the invitation-only Pace Party thrown by the dictatorial Parcells each summer in training camp at Pace University. Players were thrilled if their invitation got lost in the mail. For the first five days, each morning practice began with twenty minutes of one-on-one showdowns between the big guys on each side of the line. Parcells blew the whistle, and the players tried to destroy each other. They hated him for it. That prompted "brother-in-law" deals later in practice, when the offensive and defensive linemen took turns going easy on each other instead of smacking heads. Beginning with the first game of his rookie year in 1983, Marshall earned a spot at right defensive end with Lawrence Taylor lined up in a stand-up position to his right or behind him in the Giants 3-4 defense.

"The Pace Party. I walked around with a bottle of Tylenol the first two weeks of training camp," Marshall said. "Man-on-man, head-on-head. You knocked the living shit out of each other for twenty minutes. It wasn't fun. Trust me. Linebackers on guard. Linebackers on tight ends. Nose tackles on centers. Defensive ends on tackles. It was like a 100-mile-an-hour collision between two automobiles. Man, I hated that shit."

After the Giants drafted him in the second round from LSU, Marshall learned quickly during his rookie year that Parcells didn't have an off switch. His practices in camp were hard. He was building up his players' conditioning—physical and mental—so they would have the stamina and mental toughness to beat Washington in late-season games.

"He had worked the living shit out of me in practice one day," Marshall said.

"Put his ass back in there," Parcells screamed.

"Coach, I'm blowing the fuck out. I ain't got nothing left," Marshall said.

That was not the way to earn playing time, and Marshall knew it. He went back in. "It was my way of showing him that I got more fight in me than you will ever imagine," Marshall said. "I respected everything we did as a team because I knew there was a meaning and a purpose. I knew what doesn't kill me will make me better. I never really thought, 'Fuck them, this is about me.' It was about *we* with me. I was the perfect kind of guy to have on your team."

Marshall was not wrong. He had a career-high 15.5 sacks in 1985 and 12 the next year in the Super Bowl season. He and Taylor on the same side were a handful for the left side of any offensive line.

Players who didn't RSVP in the affirmative to the Pace Party or shied away from the physicality of training camp two-a-days discovered their luggage packed outside the dorms with one of the Giants airport drivers gassed up for the ride to LaGuardia or Newark Airport. Players were known to grab one last pop at Foley's, a neighborhood saloon around the corner from the school in suburban Pleasantville, New York, before heading to the airport.

They were asked only one question as they handed in their playbook and signed their release papers.

"Aisle or window?" Marshall said. L.T. was the Giants' superstar. Carson, Martin, and Simms were the captains. Carson considers himself "captain for life" and has gone out of his way to provide support for his ex-teammates. "Once you've won a championship, and it wasn't so much the Super Bowl game, but to go through and put the work in and do it all together, it bonds you together," Carson said. "All of those guys are my guys."

Simms, Burt, Oates, and Mark Collins were the pranksters. Simms was the heartbeat of the locker room and enjoyed holding court with the media, on and off the record. He was funny and tough, a great teammate, and a formidable practical joker. Simms and Oates went back and forth for years. Simms's go-to move was to squirt shaving cream in the pants hanging in Oates's locker and apply Vaseline to his practice cleats. "I'm ticked off after he hit me a couple of times," Oates said. Late in the 1990 season, after Simms broke his foot, he was coming in every day for treatment but not sticking around for practice. He had just bought a Jaguar from teammate Brad Benson's dealership. Oates got the keys to the car, opened the hood, took off the distributor cap, and switched around the spark plug wires.

"That messes up the timing of the car," Oates said. "It runs very rough."

From the practice field, Oates saw Simms get into his car. He was standing next to Jeff Hostetler, who had taken over at quarterback when Simms was injured.

"Hey, watch this," Oates said to Hoss.

As Simms pulled out of the parking lot, Oates could see the car shaking. Simms followed his usual path home on Route 17 North leaving the stadium. Soon the car was bucking so badly he had to pull over onto the left shoulder, creating a traffic jam and ticking off drivers, who responded by honking their horns. "Simms has a mobile phone and calls Benson and says, 'Come get this piece of crap you sold me,'" Oates said. It was a cold day with misty rain, which made it even more miserable for Simms and more satisfying for Oates. Simms was pissed. His wife picked him up, and he had the car towed to his house.

Simms brought over a mechanic to look under the hood of his expensive, brand-new car. "Somebody changed the spark plugs," he was told.

"The next morning Phil comes in, and he goes, 'I'll give a thousand bucks to whoever tells me who messed with my car yesterday,'" Oates said.

Simms knew it had to be Oates. "Bart once got in my car and put a dead fish under the seat," he said.

The stink immediately cleared out his sinuses.

"What the hell smells in here?" he said.

Simms was creative but couldn't keep up with Oates. "It was a war I couldn't win," he said. It disproved the locker-room commandment to never mess with a teammate who makes more money.

Parcells's players wouldn't recognize him these days. The first thing he does three or four mornings a week is drive to his health club to get in a workout, which he credits for still being alive after having four heart procedures, including bypass surgery, in his early fifties. Concerns about his heart led him to quit the Giants four months after winning his second Super Bowl in January 1991. He gave no explanation at the time, leaving many baffled as to why he would pass up an opportunity to repeat as champions. Long ago he stopped smoking cigarettes. He's down to just under two hundred pounds, more than fifty below his coaching weight. But even more than the slender look, Parcells's greatest transformation is his demeanor: from feared intimidator to compassionate patriarch. He hands out life advice to many of his hundreds of former players and writes life-changing checks out of the millions he has designated as his care fund for players experiencing financial distress.

He enjoys the luxury of having more money than he can spend in the golden years of his life and takes great pleasure in helping friends, among whom are his former players. "I'm really happy to see that because, oh my gosh, he was so stingy before," Burt said, laughing.

In his final two jobs coaching the Cowboys and running the front office of the Dolphins, Parcells made a total of $33 million. His four years with the Jets from 1997 to 2000, three as head coach/general manager, one as GM, earned him $10 million. There's the money he made coaching the Giants for eight years and the Patriots for four years. He's added to that with investments, endorsements, and television work with NBC and ESPN. "I got one hobby, the horses. That's not a good business. And I lose quite a bit of money every year doing that," he said.

That leads to his ex-wife questioning the wisdom of spending his money on animals he can't coach.

"What are you doing that for?" Judy Parcells said.

"Let me ask you a question: Did you go to Europe last year? You take a trip to Colorado? See your girlfriends there and stay over there at the resort?" he said.

"Yeah," she said.

"Is that your entertainment? Is that what you like?" Bill said.

"Yes," she said.

"Well, I don't do that. You take your dollars and you spend them going to Europe and I take my dollars and buy a horse. It's entertainment dollars for me," he said.

He took care of his money during his prime earning years and implored his players to take care of theirs, but he has not turned his back on those who didn't listen. He revealed he's "loaned" money to about twenty of his former players, totaling $4 million. That seems to be a conservative estimate based on the amount he mentioned he's given to some players. He said he loaned one very prominent player $2.5 million. To save the players embarrassment, he elected not to reveal names publicly. He writes the checks without the expectation of reimbursement. He does it quietly. He tries to downplay it by saying other coaches have done the same for their players, but if that is true, it's been kept completely under wraps.

Two of the Giants aware of which player received $2.5 million had differing reactions.

"It's a fucking crying shame," Phil McConkey said with disgust that the player blew his money and was so deep in the red.

"I'm surprised it's not more," George Martin said, knowing it could have been worse.

Parcells feels indebted to his former players for buying into his demanding program and risking their health and bodies for him and the team, ultimately making him a very successful coach and very rich man. He feels responsible for their well-being and wants to assist if they need money.

"They sacrificed so much for me," he said.

"A lot of guys have trouble with career transitions and a lot of them placed calls to Bill to help out," Martin said. "Bill has the means to do some things. He doesn't get the credit for it and doesn't want it. The $4 million is just the tip of the iceberg. There are so many others who need money."

Some of the '86 Giants made it big in their post-football lives. Some continue to struggle. Either way, they consider one another family. Parcells knows the inherent brutality of the NFL surely has led to the health issues, many serious, that his players have endured. If the best way to assist them is with an open checkbook policy to pay for doctors or lawyers or child support or to reduce overwhelming debt and provide peace of mind, he asks a few questions and sends the money. It's his form of philanthropy, but he first makes sure his former player really needs his money. He has embraced what he considers his responsibility.

"Why wouldn't you feel that way?" he said. "Some of these guys spent ten to twelve years with me. Some of them didn't have fathers. I feel an obligation to help them."

Banks has done very well in the business world as the president of G-III Sports, an apparel company with licensing agreements in professional and college sports. He has also managed a herniated disc in his back without requiring surgery. Carson has a sports consulting company. Simms jumped right into television after he retired in 1994 and has worked for ESPN, NBC, and CBS. Collins is an ambassador for the Kansas City Chiefs in addition to being the founder and CEO of 2FiveSports, a recruiting service for high school athletes. Gary Reasons has worked in a wide variety of fields as a college football broadcaster, an executive with Hewlett Packard Enterprise, and has helped establish telehealth for retired NFL players through the NFL Alumni Association. Pepper Johnson and Maurice Carthon had long careers as NFL assistant coaches.

Parcells had an impact on all of their lives on and off the field—and many applied the lessons he taught them in their second careers. "Bill really was a hard-ass. He knew he had to be that way to win championships," Simms said. "This is just his way of paying back the players one more time. I say one more time because he paid everybody while he was coaching by changing all of our lives. When it's all over and he sits back, he wants to reconnect with the players in a different way. He has a soft side to him, and he shows it with his generosity to a lot of his ex-players."

Simms believes that Parcells disburses the money with not one thought about getting repaid. "My dad had a great line: Never lend anybody one cent. Just give them the money. If you lend it, you will lose a friend for the rest of your life. If you give it, it will all be fine," he said.

The '86 team turned Parcells into a cult figure in New York and provided the momentum to set him up for the rest of his life. That was *the* team of his life, *the* team of their lives. He gets fifteen calls a year on Father's Day from players telling him they love him. They call him on his birthday. He calls often to check up on them and frequently ends by telling his former players he loves them.

Parcells knows that when some of the same players who call him on Father's Day call him for money, "they are desperate and only calling as the last resort," he said. "They don't have any place else to go."

One of his Giants stars has hit him up for money more than once, and the same player is into one of his teammates for $200,000. One player Parcells loved with the Patriots called him in 2022 and explained he was $60,000 short and his NFL pension wasn't kicking in for another year. Parcells hung up the phone, went to his office and wrote a check for sixty grand and put it in the mail. "I promise I will pay you back," the player said. Parcells will not send a collection agency after him if he doesn't.

This is no longer a coach-player relationship.

"I feel like a friend," Parcells said.

When he was checking up on Bavaro's health around Christmas 2021, he left a voicemail. "Hey, Mark. It's Parcells. Just calling to see how you are doing. You don't have to call me back. I love you." Bavaro has replayed the message over and over. When he played it for me at his home in Boxford, Massachusetts, he got teary-eyed. When I told Parcells how Bavaro reacted, he got teary-eyed. This goes way beyond the friendships formed as the players and coaches achieved the ultimate together in 1986. Plenty of teams win the Super Bowl. Few, if any, remain so close for so long.

This is so contrary to the relationship Parcells had with his players when he coached the Giants when many thought he was a terrible pain in the ass. He had his inner circle of "Parcells Guys" comprising Simms, Carson, Taylor, and Martin. He still coached those players hard and one time even advised Simms ahead of time he would be yelling at him at practice to get the attention of the rest of the team. But there were certainly pockets of players who didn't like him or appreciate his approach.

"I'm sure every man on that team at some point in their interactions with Bill wanted to smack him," Oates said. One former Giant said Parcells could be a "real dick." But they left it all on the field for him, and when he thought his message was not getting through, he would tell Carson to work behind the scenes in the locker room and "fix it." Carson was such an imposing man on the field with his oversized shoulder pads that the Giants sent him out as the lone captain for the Super Bowl XXI coin toss. The Broncos sent five captains. Denver won the 50–50 toss. The Giants, 9-point favorites, won 39–20. Carson wasn't just captain that season or that day. He's the first one '86 Giants teammates call when a player needs support. When backup quarterback Jeff Rutledge suffered multiple injuries in a car wreck in 2003, Carson drove seven hours from Florence, South Carolina, where he was visiting family, to where Rutledge was recuperating in Nashville. "The scary thing was going through the Smoky Mountains and its winding roads," Carson said. "But I wanted to see for myself that Jeff was okay."

Rutledge was fortunate he was alive. He was the athletic director at an all-boys school in Memphis and was driving to Nashville. He took his eyes off the road to check on a missed call on his cell phone and looked up to see an eighteen-wheeler stopped in front of him.

Rutledge was driving 65–70 miles per hour and swerved to avoid the tractor-trailer but hit a guardrail. One hour later responders were able to cut him out of his car. Rutledge was first flown back to Memphis and then to Nashville. He broke all the bones in his face, and his lip had to be sewn back on. He had brain trauma. Once he showed signs of improvement, Carson showed up unannounced to visit.

"That's the kind of guy Harry is," Rutledge said.

Aside from the accident, Rutledge has undergone back surgery and had both hips replaced. "It's tough getting old," he said. "I tell my wife, you are supposed to feel relaxed when you wake up."

Carson and Rutledge were teammates but not close friends. That didn't matter. Carson considered it his responsibility as captain to check on Rutledge, whose most noteworthy contribution in 1986 was his successful fourth-and-1 conversion off a fake punt on the Giants' first possession of the third quarter of the Super Bowl, which led to a touchdown and shifted momentum, giving New York the lead for good.

"They are Parcells's guys, but they are also my guys," Carson said. "When they hurt, I hurt. I got to find a way to ease the pain. I have a wide-ranging extensive family of guys who I love and care about. We are all part of that bond. When they say I am their captain for life, I take that literally."

Banks traces Parcells's gratitude for the sacrifices made by his players to the Giants' first practice in training camp in 1984. Parcells was coming off his disastrous three-win first season. His mother, Ida, passed away in December 1983, and his father, Charles, who played quarterback at Georgetown and was a onetime FBI agent, died six weeks later. The Giants' awful season, the illnesses of Parcells's parents, the turmoil that comes with losing, all led Young to believe the job was too big for him. If the University of Miami's Howard Schnellenberger, a close buddy of Young's from their time together with the Colts and Dolphins, had said yes to Young's offer to replace Parcells, he would have been the Giants coach in 1984. Parcells might never have been offered a second chance to be a head coach and been relegated to a life as a career assistant. But after Schnellenberger turned him down, Young told Giants owner Wellington Mara he would give Parcells one more year. If he failed, Young was confident he could get Schnellenberger in 1985. Parcells self-evaluated and concluded he lost his way making the transition from defensive coordinator to head coach. He was not being himself. His only head coaching experience had been for one season in 1978 at the Air Force Academy in Colorado Springs. This was the NFL. Assistants at any level of football—high school, college, pro—can be confidants and friends with players. Head coaches can be close to players in college. Not in professional football. Parcells needed to become a hard-ass even if it cost him friends. He had to be the boss. He knew Young would take his job if he failed.

Parcells called the players to circle around him before that first practice. "He told us they were going to fire his ass if we didn't win," Banks said. "It was as raw as can be. He was at his most vulnerable. He said, 'I cut some guys and you may not agree with that. Here is what I need from you when you make the final roster: I need to know you are my guys. I'm going to give everything I got. You give me every- thing you got.' It was the most emotional I ever saw him," Banks said, before adding a qualifier: "Other than when he had a kidney stone years later." Banks remembers it as the players going all-in, having Parcells's back, and he had theirs. "From that moment, it was just the ultimate environment of accountability and credibility," Banks said. "It set the tone for Giants football of that era. You be my guy, I'll be your guy, we are going to fight for each other. Everybody who walked through the door knew that from day one."

Parcells constantly reminded them he would have a problem with any player if his expectations for them were higher than their own. He pushed every button to help every player on the roster reach his full potential.

But Parcells could not do anything post-football to prevent Car- thon's mild stroke or William Roberts's brain tumor that fortunately turned out to be benign or Simms's severe back issues or Marshall's laundry list of aches and pains or Bavaro's struggle with long-term Covid or Bobby Johnson's hopelessness. But if Parcells could provide cash, whether it was for mortgage payments or health care, he couldn't think of a better way to use his wealth than to repay his players for their years of loyalty and dedication to him. "He's been true to that," Banks said. "It's not quid pro quo other than we all gave our best for each other. He always calls. He always checks on his guys. Every call he makes is sincere. We call and check how he is doing."

After he got out of football, Parcells set aside what he needs to live comfortably the rest of his life. He's taken care of his three daughters and ex-wife and gone as far as the tax laws allow. He took care of a grandson who needed his help. One of his former players with the Cowboys, defensive back Abe Elam, introduced him to a bright local high school senior he thought belonged in college. She came from a broken home, her father was in prison, she couldn't afford tuition, and told Parcells she would not be continuing her education after she graduated. Parcells met her and Elam for breakfast. By the time it was over, Parcells was asking her about her dream school.

"Howard University," she said.

Parcells called Jay Walker, his 1994 seventh-round draft pick for New England, who had played quarterback at Howard and worked in the school's administration. Walker told Parcells to make sure the young woman sent her documents within forty-eight hours. She was accepted right away, and Parcells picked up the full $40,000-a-year tuition for the entire four years. She graduated with excellent grades and returned to South Florida to work in the financial sector. Parcells is as proud of her as he is of any of his players.

"All this money? I never had tons of money," he said. "But I have a pretty good amount now. I give it away. That's what you do with it. When you get to my age, all I try to do is help people. You give it to your kids. You give it to your ex-wife. I give it to whoever needs it. I just try to keep enough so I can make it the rest of the way."

━━━

THE GIANTS HAVE won four Super Bowl titles; only the Patriots have won more since New York won its first in 1986. There is always something special about the first. Even though the Giants won their second Super Bowl four years later and the 2007 Giants shocked the undefeated Patriots in Super Bowl XLII and beat New England again four years later, it's the '86 team that still owns the hearts of Giants Nation. They were dominant—filled with great players, engaging personalities, a rock-star coaching staff—and broke the Giants thirty-year streak without a championship.

The first Eli Manning team that beat the Patriots in Super Bowl XLII was just 10–6 in the regular season, at the time tying for the worst record for a Super Bowl champion. Four years later they broke the record when they were 9–7 and beat the Patriots again. The 1990 team that stopped the 49ers from a three-peat and then held the Buffalo Bills fastbreak offense to just 19 points in Super Bowl XXV was resilient and resourceful but not as talented or revered as the team that won four years earlier.

In the pre–free agency days of the '70s and '80s, there was gradual improvement before a team was ready to make the final jump to a championship. You could sense when a team was building toward the Super Bowl. The sport became transient when free agency was introduced in 1993, creating small windows for teams to succeed before they enter salary cap hell and begin to lose key veterans.

That's not how it was in the '80s. In 1984, the Giants beat the Rams in the wild-card round and lost in San Francisco in the divisional round. The 49ers went on to win the Super Bowl. The following season, the Giants beat the 49ers in the wild-card round and were shut out in Chicago by the Bears in the divisional round. The Bears went on to win the Super Bowl. The Giants were convinced going into the 1986 season that it was going to be their turn. They knew to achieve their goal they not only had to win the NFC East and qualify for a first-round bye but also needed to have the best record in the NFC so their two playoff games would be at Giants Stadium.

The regular season didn't start well, as the Giants lost to the Cowboys in the season opener on Herschel Walker's 10-yard run with 1:16 left in his NFL debut, securing a 31–28 victory for Dallas. The backstory to the exciting game was that the Giants star running back Joe Morris, who had threatened not to play if he didn't have a new contract before kickoff, was speaking to his agent on a pay phone inside Texas Stadium hours before the game and was informed a four-year, $2.2 million deal had been reached. Morris rushed for a game-high 87 yards, just 2 yards fewer than Walker and Tony Dorsett combined.

The Giants won five games in a row before losing in Seattle to fall to 5–2. They didn't lose again until the opening game of the 1987 season. They won their last nine regular season games in 1986 to finish 14–2, highlighted by Bobby Johnson's fourth-and-17 sideline grab to set up the winning field goal in Minnesota and a memorable catch and run by Bavaro carrying virtually the entire 49ers defense—and overwhelmed Washington, San Francisco, and Denver by a combined 105–23 in the playoffs.

Wire to wire, the '86 Giants had the look of a Super Bowl champion.

—————

NOT ENOUGH PLAYERS worry about life after football in real time. In the moment, they think they are Superman dressed in a football jersey, when football is chock full of kryptonite.

CTE? Not me. I only had my "bell rung" a few times.

Knee replacement? Not with all the weight training.

Excruciating back pain? Ah, just take a couple of Advil, right?

Heart issues? Finishing first in the training camp conditioning runs? It ensures nothing. Better look up the meaning of ablation.

Ninety-five percent of NFL players are replaceable parts coming off an assembly line. It's a world of next man up. That's why they don't ever want to come off the field, fearing they will lose their job. Football careers are often over before college classmates finish up their law degree or MBA. The locker room motto: Can't make the club in the tub. The best ability is availability. That has led to a barbaric culture in the NFL. The average career lasts 3.3 years. Anything more is wishful thinking. Tom Brady is a once-in-a-century phenomenon. The earning potential for today's players has become outrageous, even for the fifty-third man on the roster, but it's over a limited number of years. In this era of the NFL, players can set themselves up financially for life in 3.3 years, but the money for the players in the 1980s who made it to their fourth year was not life changing.

Would the '86 Giants do it all over again knowing what they know now about the long-term damage the game has done to their bodies? The game allowed them to be part of an incredible championship, and for some it's given them financial independence. For others, the physical price they've paid is overwhelming and not worth it.

"Given what I know now, if I had to do it all over again, I would not have done it," Carson said.

"At the end of the day, I wouldn't trade it," Taylor said.

Then he thinks about the aches and pains in his sixties. And perhaps he thinks if he didn't play football he never would have had the resources to become addicted to cocaine.

He paused for a moment.

"Would I trade it?" he said. "Maybe. I don't know."

═══

IN RECONNECTING WITH the '86 Giants, I wanted to hear the fun boys-will-be-boys behind-the-scenes account of their glorious season and how they produced this brotherhood for eternity. The exhausting journey to a championship created an unbreakable bond from the top of the roster to the bottom. But it was also crucial to chronicle life after football and not only for marquee players such as Taylor, Simms, Carson, Banks, Bavaro, Morris, and Marshall but the support group of Bobby Johnson, McConkey, Karl Nelson, William Roberts, Maurice Carthon, Mark Collins, Curtis McGriff, Pepper Johnson, Reasons, Oates, and others.

What's life been like since they removed their helmets for the last time? Instead of cherry-picking players around the NFL in the '80s, it was more compelling to select one team, a championship team, the most popular team in the history of one of the NFL's cornerstone franchises in the greatest city in the world, whose experience summarizes for every man who has ever played in the NFL the challenges presented by life after football.

The '86 Giants illustrate the unbeatable formula when talent, dedication, leadership, and Hall of Fame coaching collide.

The locker-room stories and practical jokes are hilarious.

The sad stories are compelling and tragic.

"I thought my generation and my group of players was going to avoid it, and I was wrong," Simms said. "I just thought we had progressed a little further along and knew a little bit more about taking care of ourselves, and we wouldn't be all crippled when we were sixty years old. Every generation that comes along, we are better than the group before us. But it's not as dramatic as I thought it would be."

The physical toll of playing football is so severe that Reasons, a linebacker, calls himself a "freak of nature" because he's never had major surgery, never had cognitive issues, and has no physical problems after playing nine years in the NFL. "I've come through pretty clean," he said. "The game is so nasty. It's difficult. Most guys come away hindered in some capacity."

Life after football for the 1986 Giants has been heartwarming and heartbreaking.

"The thing I am most proud of this group for is they are still a team," Parcells said. "If one of them is in trouble, the others show up. That is what a team is supposed to be."

As I traveled to meet in person or spoke on the phone with the players and coaches, their stories were beyond my expectations. Four players contemplated suicide *after* football. Carson also described how a few years into his Giants career, he was so depressed he got into his car on the way to work at Giants Stadium and gave serious thought to steering off the westbound Tappan Zee Bridge into the Hudson River.

One player's back pain was so severe twenty years and three major surgeries after he last played, he downed a potentially dangerous combination of straight vodka with a painkiller to provide temporary relief. My long-term relationships with so many of the Giants players, established by covering their games and staying in touch after their careers ended, allowed me to approach the project with built-in trust, which led to forthcoming conversations on sensitive topics. Heart-warming or heartbreaking, names will be attached to stories, except in the few cases when a player requested anonymity to avoid embarrassing himself or a teammate.

Belichick was extraordinarily cooperative in providing insight for this book, even though he rarely contributes to outside projects. He loved the 1986 team and once texted Carson to thank him for looking out for his teammates.

Belichick received his second opportunity to be a head coach when he was hired by the Patriots in 2000. He drafted Brady in the sixth round that year, and they went on to win six Super Bowls together. Along with the two he won with the Giants in his twelve seasons in New York, Belichick has eight Super Bowl rings. His accomplishments in New England make him the greatest coach in NFL history as he closes in on Don Shula's all-time record for victories, but his foundation was set with the Giants. And he is both melancholy and appreciative of his time in New York and how that group helped advance his career.

"I keep in touch with quite a few of them," he said. "Unfortunately, some of them are not doing so well; others are doing very well. Harry came over to talk to our team before the New York Giants preseason game in 2021. We caught up for quite a while. I probably see five to seven of them a year. I have missed a couple of reunions that took place during the season, but I always enjoy seeing the pictures. Most of those players text me after a big win, and I certainly appreciate hearing from them."

The 1986 season was a fairy tale for the Giants. But in real life, not everyone lives happily ever after. This book is the story of what really happens after the confetti stops falling and the special bond between the players who helped one another survive it.

They had one another's backs every Sunday. They also took care of one another when they put their helmets and shoulder pads in their lockers after practice and hit the streets to take advantage of being sports celebrities in New York.

PART I

WORK HARD, PLAY HARD

1

DON'T SLEEP ON THE GIANTS

The world's most decadent amusement park for the rich and famous in the mid-1980s was eight miles from Giants Stadium: New York City. On Friday nights during the 1986 season, the rich and famous New York Giants made the short trip from East Rutherford and hit the streets ready to party at the end of another week of practice. They were welcomed at the door by bouncers at the hottest clubs and invited to cut the line.

Step right in, Big Blue.

"The city loved us," Carl Banks said. "It was just a fun, fun time. Just being part of the fabric as a group, part of the fabric of New York, just doing stuff together, it was a lot of fun."

Studio 54, Nell's, the Palladium, China Club, the Hard Rock Cafe.

The women were plentiful, the booze flowed freely, and cocaine was readily available in the back rooms. The NFL didn't begin its drug-testing program until 1987, and even to this day it contains a major loophole. Once a player passed the annual mandatory urine test, he was off the hook until the following summer. Only if he gave the team reasonable cause to believe he was snorting coke or smoking crack or weed was a player subjected to random testing.

It was no secret around the Giants that Lawrence Taylor had an out-of-control cocaine problem. He finally checked into a rehab center in Houston for the first time in March 1986, not that it did much good. His life was filled with sacks on the field and cocaine off it, and his dedication to drugs didn't prevent him from dominating and intimidating on Sundays.

"In the past year, due to substance abuse, I have left the road that I had hoped to follow both as a player and as a public figure," Taylor said when he got out of rehab. "In recent months, I have privately sought professional assistance to help me with these problems. I have just completed the first phase in what I know will be a difficult and ongoing battle to overcome these problems."

Nine months later, Taylor was named NFL MVP and Defensive Player of the Year after a career-high 20.5 sacks. During the team's championship run, he was a wrecking ball.

The doors of New York's hottest night spots swung open for the Giants as the lines stretched around the corner and down the block. They were good for business, along with the recently crowned World Series champion Mets, baseball's version of Animal House, and they were often out clubbing together. The guys at the bars lined up to talk with the Giants. The ladies often wanted something more, not that the feeling wasn't mutual. Giants Stadium might have been built on swampland and surrounded by diners and fast-food joints, but city life beckoned just a half hour away.

For Taylor, every night was a night to play. He caught up on sleep at Giants Stadium in team meetings.

"It was not uncommon for players to go out in groups," Banks said. "It was a circuit we would all do. And at some point, we would run into Lawrence. It might have been at Nell's, which didn't close until seven in the morning." Nell's was such a big deal that the *New York Times* led its Style section with a piece titled "The Mighty Nell's."

The Giants on the circuit put together a busy agenda. They would shower and leave the locker room after Friday practice, dressed and ready to head into the night. "A group of us were really snazzy dressers," Banks said.

Pregaming on Friday nights during the season was in New Jersey before the players crossed the river into Manhattan. There was Joey's in Clifton up Route 3 from the stadium, a favorite spot of wide receiver Lionel Manuel, the recipient of Simms's first pass in the Super Bowl. Banks often liked to get warmed up at Club Zanzibar in Newark. Banks, Pepper Johnson, and Elvis Patterson discovered a skating rink to do a few laps to unwind in Teaneck close to the George Washington Bridge, which provided easy access to the FDR Drive and West Side Highway once rush hour traffic subsided.

Bill Parcells conducted 9 a.m. meetings on Saturdays at the stadium, but that didn't discourage a significant number of Giants from pulling all-nighters like they were back in college.

If the Giants were playing at home, they had Saturday afternoon off to nap before reporting to the Hilton Woodcliff Lake, the team hotel, fifteen miles north of the stadium, where they were required to stay. If they were on the road, they caught up on sleep on the flight. A curfew curtailed partying the night before games, home and away, unless a player wanted to risk getting caught and fined. That happened all the time in training camp. Not as much during the regular season, although Bobby Johnson's quest for crack and female companionship led him over the wall the night before the 17–0 victory over Washington in the 1986 NFC Championship Game, showing up in the locker room minutes before kickoff. If the Giants were playing on the road, players left their cars in the stadium parking lot after Saturday's walk-through and took the team bus to Newark Airport, which dropped them off on the tarmac next to their chartered flight.

Football life is structured. Meetings and practice times vary slightly from day to day. It's a regimen that players are accustomed to since high school, and a good many of them embrace the discipline it instills. It's the hours away from the field that worry coaches. They live in fear of the 2 a.m. phone call from the team security director or the local police that one of their players has been arrested for driving drunk on the George Washington Bridge or has fallen asleep on the shoulder of the New Jersey Turnpike or Garden State Parkway. Giants coach Tom Coughlin and GM Jerry Reese received a call the night after Thanksgiving in 2008 that star wide receiver Plaxico Burress had shot himself in the leg while walking up the stairs at the Latin Quarter, an East Side club, nearly ten months after catching the winning touchdown in Super Bowl XLII. Burress was packing heat for protection and had it tucked in the waistband of his sweatsuit when it inadvertently fired, forcing him to miss the rest of the season and ruining the team's chances to repeat as Super Bowl champions. The gun was not registered in New York, and it cost Burress twenty-two months in prison. When he returned to the field in 2011, he was no longer a Giant, no longer remembered as a Super Bowl hero, and his skills had diminished.

On Friday nights during the 1986 season, once the players left the building, they were on their own until the Saturday morning meeting. They lived for Friday nights but faced a logistical dilemma in the few hours between leaving the clubs at 4 a.m. and the start of Parcells's meeting. Oversleeping the team meeting was not an option, and being tardy for the team flight was the equivalent of begging Parcells to get cut.

The solution was much easier than blocking Reggie White or devising a scheme to sack Randall Cunningham. The partiers simply skipped going home Friday night and went right from the city to the players' parking lot at Giants Stadium to sleep in their cars. The parking lot was multipurpose. L.T., with his Porsche, often raced Brad Benson, to the delight of teammates. At least they had the good sense to race during weekday business hours when the lot was empty and not stage the Meadowlands 500, considering all the light posts that needed to be avoided.

After a long Friday night, at 4:30 a.m. Saturday, there was a parade of headlights entering Lot 9 on the west side of the stadium. At 8:55 a.m., there was a parade of tired football players walking twenty-five yards down the ramp into the stadium and then turning left and left again and sleepwalking their way into Parcells's meeting.

The '86 crew was resourceful. When they partied until they could party no more, no matter how late, the system they devised kept them punctual. They took their after-hours bar-hanging and bar-hopping seriously, but the '86 Giants knew it was their year to win the Super Bowl, so football was still high up on their priority list. They didn't want to look back and regret leaving their best moves on the dance floor or in dark corners at the China Club or Nell's.

Banks enlisted the help of locker room manager Kevin Croke, the son of Giants longtime public relations director Ed Croke, to organize a group of ambitious locker room attendants looking to make some money on the side to go from car to car at 8:45 a.m. waking up players too hungover to arise on their own.

"I never knew about that," Parcells said. "If they missed a meeting, and it didn't happen much, they were fined a lot of money."

Croke and his crew were not allowed to take "get the fuck out of here" for an answer from their clients. They were not to return to the locker room without bringing a player with them. Cell phones with alarms were still only on *The Jetsons*, so the locker room kids were the last line of defense. Croke was a favorite of the veterans. At training camp, he would alert them "when the dorm was clear of coaches" doing bed check, Banks said. "He was an ally of ours so we could sneak out."

The parking lot system was well thought out.

"We had a group of ball boys who were assigned to specific players," Banks said. "The ball boys would knock on the windows of the cars when it was time to go to the meeting. Some guys who didn't sleep in their cars didn't show up for meetings and didn't make the plane. That used to piss off Bill, and it pissed us off, too. That's why we came up with this system. Whenever we were finished in the city, we were not allowed to go home. We would go straight to the stadium parking lot."

It was a cost-efficient program. The charge for the wake-up call was $50 for each player, a nominal fee considering the four-figure fines they avoided. Coffee, orange juice, and toothbrushes were not included as part of the concierge service. Late to bed and early to rise was a successful formula for the '86 Giants. "I didn't know about them sleeping in their cars," said punter Sean Landeta, who had many female companions in Manhattan but didn't use his car as an apartment. "If you're late, you get fined thousands of dollars. So it was very smart on their part."

If the Giants were playing on the road, the Friday nightclub crew packed travel clothes and tossed their bags into the trunk of their cars. The players drove themselves into the city or carpooled; the smart ones enlisted a limousine service to navigate, eliminating any possibility of getting stopped for driving while intoxicated.

"This was part of our whole bond—solving problems for each other and making sure we can all be accountable and not letting each other down," Banks said.

The Giants looked out for each other in the city, which translated into looking out for each other on Sunday afternoons. Many of them lived close to the stadium, in Clifton and Secaucus or in Hoboken, just on the Jersey side of the Lincoln Tunnel. Some lived thirty minutes away in Franklin Lakes or Upper Saddle River. Regardless of their proximity, arriving in the parking lot at 4:30 a.m. rather than going home gave them a much better opportunity to be on time for work.

Banks lived in Secaucus, only two and a half miles from the parking lot. Nell's, a converted electronics store, was his favorite spot. It was on West Fourteenth Street and opened in the fall of 1986. "The earliest anybody ever leaves Nell's is 3:30, 4 o'clock in the morning," Banks said. "On any given night if we're there, there's Mike Tyson, Darryl Strawberry, there's Doc [Dwight Gooden], there's Keith Hernandez. It's literally a who's who. There's Madonna. You just party. Dance."

And then drive to Giants Stadium. And go to sleep. In the parking lot.

———

LANDETA WAS A legend in the Giants locker room, and it had nothing to do with Phil Simms declaring, "He's the greatest punter in NFL history and I don't think it's an argument."

Even better than Ray Guy, Simms said, who is the only punter in the Pro Football Hall of Fame. Unfortunately for Landeta, too many football fans remember him for "the whiff," when the swirling winds at a frigid Soldier Field blew the ball away from his right foot and he missed it completely on a punt attempt from the Giants' 12-yard line in the first quarter of a 21–0 divisional round playoff loss in 1985. Shaun Gayle scooped up the loose ball for the Bears and returned it five yards for an easy touchdown to give Chicago a 7–0 lead.

Parcells asked Landeta what happened when he came to the sideline. Landeta told him he missed the ball. They never spoke about it again. "When you watch the tape, you can see the wind knocked the ball away," Parcells said. But proving he was still unforgiving so many decades later, he added, "That shouldn't happen. You should make some kind of contact with it."

Landeta's swing and miss may be an NFL original and a regular on blooper shows, but the truth is, the Giants had no chance to win that game anyway because they were never going to score enough against the best defense in NFL history. "An ass whooping," Taylor said.

Even so, the Giants trailed by only 7–0 when they had a first-and-goal at the Bears' 2-yard line with twenty-nine seconds remaining in the first half. Simms tossed three straight incompletions before Eric Schubert hit the left upright on a chip-shot 19-yard field goal attempt. The Bears scored their second touchdown six minutes into the third quarter, and the game was over.

Schubert was kicking for the Cardinals the next season. At least Parcells held onto his punter.

The affable Landeta is still sensitive about the mishap. "It was just a bad moment and bad luck. That's all it was. The wind just moved the drop as I went to punt it. There's no definitive explanation," he said. "My teammates realized it was just a fluke play. But if this is about the '86 Giants, why are you asking me about that play from the year before?"

It's all part of the Landeta legacy.

"We could have killed that guy when he missed that punt," said Taylor, who now considers Landeta one of his best friends from the '86 team.

Landeta redeemed himself in the NFC Championship Game the following year by being the best player on the field. Even Taylor acknowledged Landeta won the game, and L.T. considered punters one step above the league's urine collectors. Landeta was an artist in the way he mastered the winds that gusted to 25 miles per hour at Giants Stadium. He averaged over 42 yards per punt and won the field position battle for the Giants in their shutout victory over Washington.

"Every time I see Sean Landeta, I tell him he was the MVP of that game," Taylor said. "Without him and what he did . . . ," Taylor's voice trails off. It must kill him to praise a punter. "He made up for the previous year," he said.

Whether Landeta is the GOAT of punters is a reasonable debate, but he was unquestionably the GOAT of New York Giants nightlife. A punter on a team with All-Pro players/partiers outdid them all with the ladies.

"He was a character and I loved him," said Phil McConkey, a wide receiver and punt returner. "I remember going to Simms and saying, 'Yeah, he's a football player, but he's a punter. He's kind of a pudgy punter. How does he get all these girls?'"

Simms was married, so he just got a kick out of Landeta's exploits. McConkey was single, and although the New York club scene was certainly big enough for the two of them, he was perplexed at Landeta's success rate. During one game, as McConkey came off the field after a mundane 4-yard punt return, he said Landeta came up to him and started raving how he was the best in the league catching punts. "He was a great teammate," McConkey said.

In return for all the compliments, one teammate scouted women in the bleachers at training camp for Landeta as they stood together making sure the defensive players touched the line as they ran gassers.

"Look at her. *Holy shit*," the player said. "You got to see this girl. She's the prettiest girl I've ever seen at camp."

Landeta turned his head.

"I'm glad you said that," Landeta said. "That's the girl I'm dating." Next.

McConkey believed Landeta's schtick was relatively transparent. He came to that conclusion after Landeta praised his punt catching skills.

"Simms, I got this guy figured out. I got it nailed," McConkey said. "What do women want? Praise that makes them feel good. He tells you that you are the greatest quarterback ever. He's making these women feel that way. That was the secret."

Landeta had an endearing way about him that made every woman feel like a beauty pageant queen. (In many cases, they were.) He was a positive person, and it paid off well for him on the circuit, even if he was a pudgy punter. He signed with the Giants in 1985 after three years with the Philadelphia/Baltimore Stars in the USFL and became best friends with veteran punter Dave Jennings, his competition in training camp. Jennings was a fan favorite and one of the most popular Giants among his teammates. Besides being an excellent punter, Jennings was responsible for the NFL creating statistics for punts inside the 20 and net yardage, which was a much better indication of a punter's effectiveness than total distance, which rewarded booming punts that resulted in touchbacks. Landeta was ten years younger than Jennings and had a stronger leg and won the job, but Jennings still treated him like his little brother, even after Jennings was cut and signed with the Jets.

Jennings, who died from Parkinson's disease at the age of sixty-one in 2013, punted eleven seasons for the Giants and three more for the Jets and helped Landeta feel at home in New York. He kept his house in Upper Saddle River. Although the Jets played at Giants Stadium, their practice facility was on Long Island, a solid seventy-five-minute drive on a good day. Landeta would stop by Jennings's house after work to watch *Monday Night Football*. "Dave was so good to me," he said. "He could have been a real dick, but he was so gracious."

One bit of kindness by Jennings created a clear path for Landeta to the red carpet of New York City.

"Dave introduced me to his longtime dear friend Sy Presten," he said.

Presten, who died in 2022 at the age of ninety-eight, was a throwback to the days of New York public relations power brokers. He invited Jennings, who was single, friendly, and media conscious, to many high-profile events over the years. On Jennings's say-so, Landeta was added to Presten's exclusive invitation list.

Landeta was just twenty-three years old in his first season with the Giants and would be named first team punter on the All-Decade Team of the 1980s and second team on the 1990s team.

But he was first team on a list that made his teammates jealous.

Landeta was first-team All-Penthouse.

Presten got him on a list to die for.

One of Presten's clients was the adult magazine *Penthouse*. If *Playboy* was rated for mature audiences, then *Penthouse* was X-rated. *Penthouse* was owned by Bob Guccione, who was also the proprietor of a seven-story townhouse on Sixty-Seventh Street between Madison Avenue and Fifth Avenue on the East Side of Manhattan. It was the answer to Hugh Hefner's Playboy Mansion in Los Angeles, a favorite of Dallas Cowboys players who broke curfew in the '80s when their training camp was held in Thousand Oaks, California.

Guccione's palace had an elevator, expensive art, and a swimming pool on the second floor. "Don't get too close to the artwork," Landeta said. "If you breathe on it, the alarm goes off." Light mood music played in the background. Landeta worked himself onto the regular guest list whenever Guccione was throwing a party. Landeta couldn't help but be surrounded by beautiful women.

"I had a chance to meet a number of girls, and they were all very nice," he said.

Presten proved to be an invaluable liaison for Landeta as he dated Penthouse Pets after meeting them at the parties. He once looked around Guccione's townhouse and realized he was the only New York athlete in attendance. How did that happen? No quarterbacks from the

Giants or Jets; no pitchers, shortstops, or centerfielders from the Mets or Yankees; no shooting guards from the Knicks or high-scoring right wings from the Rangers. It had to be a dream. Landeta was a punter. Really, how the hell did that happen?

"I owe it all to Dave Jennings," he said.

Landeta told the *Baltimore Sun* in 1991, "I'm not afraid to admit that if I wasn't playing pro football, there's no way I could have dated some of the girls I did. They were way too pretty for me. I think back to some of them, and it's like, geez."

That's exactly what his teammates were thinking. Good-natured teasing of Landeta was another bonding experience in the locker room.

Landeta was on the gossip pages of the New York tabloids more than the sports pages. He was a star of Page Six in the *New York Post*. "I was just a single guy playing in the NFL," he said. "I didn't drink, smoke, do drugs, gamble, or go to strip joints. I had to do something." Landeta still claims his active social life was exaggerated. "Every time I went out with a girl, like most every other single player would, it would be in the newspaper," he said. "So, the perception was much greater than the reality."

Maybe.

Maybe not.

"Maybe the fact that a few of them had a title next to their name had something to do with it," he said.

Beauty pageant winners and Penthouse Pets have titles before their names. Miss USA. Miss April.

"I don't recall the titles," Landeta said, laughing. "You date a girl who might have been a model, the papers make more out of it than they should have."

Jim Burt went to a baseball game at Yankee Stadium with Landeta, and they sat behind the Yankees dugout. He had an opportunity to observe Landeta's magic ways up close. "I witnessed it firsthand," Burt said. "He had a big old beer belly, and I just don't know how he did it. We were sitting at the game, and he just looked over at a girl and she comes over. Then another girl comes over. Then he's leaving with a bunch of girls in a limousine. I went stage left. I'm out of here. I was married. He was a freaking magnet. Sean Lan-freaking-deta."

Landeta knew if his picture appeared in the front section of the tabloids, he would immediately get teased by his teammates. It gave him unlimited street cred in the locker room. "They didn't want to hear it, but I told them, 'I'm not doing anything you're not,'" he said. "It was the '80s, just that time in our society, it was a booming decade. And we were doing so well as a team. There was just so many things to do. A lot of guys were out a lot more than me. I guarantee you that."

McConkey did his best to catch up to Landeta but suffered a huge setback when Parcells cut him on the Monday before the '86 season opener in Dallas. He was claimed on waivers by the Packers. All of Green Bay could fit into Nell's. Fortunately for McConkey's career and social life, Giants wide receiver Lionel Manuel sprained his knee in the fourth game of the season against the Saints. He had been splitting the punt returning with cornerback Mark Collins. Parcells needed a receiver, and McConkey was a better punt returner than Collins. McConkey represented two for the price of one. He was watching film at the Packers office at Lambeau Field when he was told that Packers coach Forrest Gregg wanted to see him in his office the day after Manuel was hurt.

"Bring your playbook," he was told.

The three words players never want to hear. It usually precedes, "Thanks, but we're going in a different direction. Here's your plane ticket."

Aisle or window?

"We traded you back to the Giants," Gregg said.

"You got to be kidding me," is all McConkey could think to say.

Thank you also would have been appropriate.

McConkey was elated. Gregg had to run to a staff meeting but told him to wait in his office for Parcells to call. He had been in Green Bay just four weeks, not nearly long enough to get attached to his teammates, embraced by the fans, discover the charm of living in the smallest city in the league, or become the Landeta of the Green Bay circuit. He never wanted to leave the Giants and thought Parcells made a mistake cutting him.

McConkey sat in Gregg's office. The phone rang. The voice was familiar.

"Hey, McConkey, those Packers drive a hard bargain," Parcells said.

"What are you talking about?" McConkey said.

"I had to throw in a couple clipboards with a blocking dummy to get you back. That's what you're worth. So, get your ass over here and catch some punts," Parcells said.

Parcells traded a twelfth-round draft pick to the Packers, a round that doesn't exist anymore and might have had less value than a clipboard and blocking dummy.

Parcells asked him what it was like in Green Bay.

"The grass is greener, my ass," McConkey said.

"Listen, when you get in, I want you to write that on the chalkboard in the locker room," Parcells said.

It was a reminder to the rest of the team that regardless how hard Parcells worked them or how much they would have enjoyed stuffing him in a locker, they were better off with the devil they knew than the devil they didn't know, especially if the perceived devil was coaching a Super Bowl contender.

McConkey did as he was asked and scribbled "The Grass Is Greener, My Ass" on the chalkboard at the entrance to the Giants locker room, and his words remained all season. McConkey would have walked from Green Bay to New York if that was the only way. Not only was he back where he wanted to be, but his social life took a turn for the much better.

McConkey went to college at the Naval Academy, fulfilled his five-year commitment after graduation, and decided it was time to give up his commission and move into civilian life. He was an accomplished helicopter pilot who suffered from motion sickness, which is not an ailment conducive to a lifetime career in the navy.

Long-time US Naval Academy assistant coach and scout Steve Belichick recommended him to his son Bill, who was coaching linebackers and special teams for the Giants. The team invited him to a rookie minicamp with their draft picks and rookie free agents. McConkey had written a letter to Norm Pollom, the director of player personnel for his hometown Buffalo Bills, and was hoping to get a tryout with them as well. As McConkey was stretching for the afternoon practice on the second of three days of two-a-days with the rookies, Parcells asked him why he hadn't yet signed the contract the Giants offered. Still hoping to hear from the Bills, McConkey stumbled a bit with his answer, so Parcells added $1,000 to his $10,000 signing bonus to go along with the $55,000 base salary and incentives. McConkey set his Bills dreams aside and signed the deal. He made $100,000 his rookie season.

"I would have given them $100,000," McConkey said. "I'd have signed my life away to play for the New York Giants and play in the NFL."

He was twenty-seven years old when he showed up at Giants camp in 1984, and he was one month short of his thirtieth birthday when he caught a long flea-flicker and later scored a touchdown in the Super Bowl. He was 5'10", not even 160 pounds, and looked more like a financial advisor, which he is today, but he was a tough little guy who proved to be an invaluable member of a Super Bowl championship team. Roger Staubach, the former Navy and Cowboys quarterback, was McConkey's hero. He still reveres him, and they've become friends. A few days after the Super Bowl, there was an autographed picture in the mail from Staubach with the inscription, "From one USNA Super Bowl champion to another."

He was also an unlikely star of the nightclub circuit. His big night was Monday, which preceded the weekly Tuesday players' day off.

Before McConkey became a Super Bowl hero, he used to patronize the Hard Rock Cafe in the city with Mark Bavaro, who showed up with torn jeans, sneakers with no laces, and a Boston Celtics tank top. "He had muscles on muscles," McConkey said. "He had long hair and five or six days' worth of growth. He didn't give two shits about the way he looked. I remember girls just swooning. Mark was totally oblivious."

Bavaro was soon to be married and was just interested in hanging out. Once McConkey became a recognizable face, the city opened up to him. "Monday night at the China Club in the '80s was epic," McConkey said. "You go down these steps and there was a rectangular bar with a fish tank with mini-sharks. Behind the bar was a dance floor with a little stage. And to the left of that they had a VIP section."

Two or three off-duty New York City cops would guard the VIP area popular with celebrities, athletes, and models. McConkey usually met up with his friend Keith Hernandez of the Mets. Elton John, Bruce Springsteen, the O'Jays, or the Fifth Dimension would appear and do a set on stage. Even though Tuesday was his day off, McConkey set a self-imposed 11 p.m. curfew just as the China Club shifted into second gear.

That didn't exclude him from the high-octane nightlife. Good things can still happen before 11. He was amazed at baseball players' capacity to party deep into the night. "I mean, football players are crazy, but baseball players are out of their minds," he said. "At least football players had to go to practice the next day and they drank and maybe did some drugs, but those guys didn't have to get up the next day. They played [their games] at night. They were night owls."

McConkey was approached by celebrities, models, and athletes and invited to join them in the small office to the left of the bar. It was dark, cramped, and hot in there. He was hanging with the girls, listening to the music, and nursing his one beer or margarita that took him until his curfew. "What do I want to go to the office for?" he said. Everything he came to the China Club for was on the dance floor. Why leave the pretty ladies? "I didn't know until much later on that they were going to the office to do cocaine," he said. "I had no clue. They must have thought I was from another planet."

His father was a cop in Buffalo. He spent nearly a decade with the navy between school and his commitment. "I always thought if I did drugs, my heart would pop right out of my chest," he said. "I was terrified."

=====

HARRY CARSON WAS a legend in the locker room for his prowess with women. During breaks in practice is when Carson would share stories with teammates. They listened with great admiration. "Harry was famous for kissing and telling," Banks said.

"I want to emphasize I was single," Carson said.

He didn't drink or do drugs. He never got into trouble off the field. He also wasn't married until June 25, 1988, one month before training camp of his final year in the league. He got divorced after about ten years and later married his current wife, Maribel. But for his first twelve years in the league, he was one of New York's most eligible bachelors.

One offseason he worked at Grumman Aerospace in Bethpage on Long Island and invited a woman he met there to visit him in training camp. She stopped by on the same day another woman he was dating came to see him, and Carson enlisted one of his teammates to cover for him with one of them.

"I remember Parcells saying you should be one of those UN ambassadors because you don't discriminate," Carson said. "I didn't discriminate. I dated Black women, I dated white women, I dated Latino women, I dated Asian women. And so that was my only weakness. I was single so I could do whatever I wanted. Once I got married, that was a different story."

A very different story, indeed.

He met a woman in 1979 when he was in Chicago during the offseason, and they stayed in touch. Carson saw on the schedule the Giants were playing the Chiefs in Kansas City on October 21 and invited his new friend to make the short trip from Chicago so they could spend time together. The Giants, as usual, arrived in town the day before the game. Carson said his social life never impacted football except for that game in Kansas City. He was very tired on game day after a busy Saturday night, and to make it worse, it was a very hot day. "I was winded," he said. "I made a deal with God. I said, 'God, if you get me out of this, I'll never do it again.'"

New York trailed 17–14, and the Chiefs were trying to run out the clock with less than two minutes left. On a second and 6 from the Kansas City 22-yard line, quarterback Mike Livingston handed off to running back Mike Williams. Carson's pal Brian Kelley greeted Williams and stuck in his right hand, forcing a fumble. Carson picked up the loose ball on one hop and ran it 22 yards for the winning touchdown with 1:42 left in the game.

Carson was happy to get out of Kansas City with a victory. It was the Giants' third straight after a 0–5 start. After Carson showered and dressed, his lady friend was waiting for him by the team bus taking them to the airport for the flight home. She needed a ride to the airport for her flight back to Chicago. Giants owner Wellington Mara, a devoted family man, was standing nearby.

"Mr. Mara," Carson said, "this is my cousin. Can we give her a ride to the airport?"

Mara was in a good mood after the victory and particularly happy with Carson after he scored the winning touchdown.

"Harry, you know you can have anything you want," Mara said.

Carson and his friend sat in the first row behind the bus driver. They were holding hands. Mara was directly across the aisle and took note. When the woman was dropped off at the terminal to catch her flight and the Giants were driving another couple of minutes to get to their charter, Mara looked over to Carson.

"I understand how cousins can be very close," Mara said. "But I didn't realize they could be *that close*."

One of the reasons Carson didn't go into coaching was because he knew how players behaved on the road, and he didn't want his job depending on them. The Giants played in St. Louis every year, and it didn't take Carson long to figure out during his rookie year that many of his teammates had a woman they would meet when they got into town.

"I'm like, damn, you know, this is going to be pretty nice," he said.

Ed Croke, the Giants public relations director, would arrive in the visiting city on Tuesday before the game to brief the opposing team's media and set up all the logistical details at the team hotel for the Giants' arrival on Saturday. If Carson had a weekend visitor, he would request Croke give him a room at the end of the hallway. Players did not have single rooms, so Croke would set aside another room for Carson's guest also at the end of the hall one floor above or below his room, making it easier to sneak out after curfew.

"That was part of the reason why we probably weren't all that good during those down years," Carson said.

———

FOOTBALL PLAYERS SPEND more than six months together from the start of training camp until the end of the season. They see each other at least six out of the seven days during the week. They come up with practical jokes to keep from going crazy. But when practical jokes turn into hazing or have a cruel intent, it can cause friction. Locker room humor can be brutal.

Hazing has become virtually nonexistent in the NFL. The days of tying a rookie up to the goalpost after practice and pouring honey on him to attract bees are over. It doesn't get much worse now than forcing a rookie to sing his school fight song in the cafeteria at lunchtime (though even that has led to fighting, including a 2002 shoving match involving Giants rookie tight end Jeremy Shockey and veteran linebacker Brandon Short). When Carson tried to get rookie tight end Mark Bavaro to sing the Notre Dame fight song in 1985, he refused. Bavaro was very quiet, and the vets didn't know what to make of him. Instead of pushing it with him more than a time or two, Carson backed off.

Mark Collins's signature trick was an all-time favorite that never fails. The carpet in the Giants locker room was in the team colors: blue and red. Collins took a $100 bill out of his pocket, poked a tiny hole in it and threaded a piece of black shoestring through it to blend into the carpet. Wide receiver Stacy Robinson was his lookout and would signal Collins when a sucker was coming around the corner. As soon as his target bent down to pick up the free money, Collins pulled the string.

"I got everybody," Collins said proudly. "I got Parcells."

"Damn you, Collins," Parcells barked.

Collins loved strength coach Johnny Parker.

"He fell for it five times," Collins said. "How can you fall for this five times?"

Bavaro and McConkey were best friends and roommates for road games. Bavaro's former Giants teammate and mentor Don Hasselbeck was vacationing in Hawaii and sent him a box of chocolate-covered macadamia nuts, a Bavaro favorite. The night before a big game in 1986, Bavaro opened the box of nuts in the hotel and was popping them in his mouth one after the other. McConkey noticed that some of the chocolate on the nuts had turned white, which McConkey knew was harmless. He also knew Bavaro was always complaining about stomach issues.

"You didn't eat those, did you?" McConkey asked.

"Why?" Bavaro said.

"The white coating. You can't eat that," McConkey said with a grave voice and serious face.

McConkey took a knife and cut through the chocolate and the nut.

"Oh, shit," he said.

"Why? What's the big deal?" Bavaro asked.

"You don't know what that is? It's *Fungi bartoli*," McConkey said.

McConkey went on for two minutes about how Bavaro was going to get violently ill from *Fungi bartoli*, a fungus he just made up that caused major stomach problems in twelve to twenty-four hours—just in time for kickoff. Bavaro panicked. Oh shit, *Fungi bartoli*. How was he going to tell Parcells he had this dreaded malady and couldn't play doubled over in the bathroom? Bavaro immediately called the hotel operator to connect him to trainer Ronnie Barnes's room.

"I started crying," Bavaro said.

McConkey had already called Barnes imploring him to play along. "Ronnie was in on it for a little while," McConkey said. "Of course, Ronnie is such a nice guy he couldn't keep it going. He couldn't tell a lie if his life depended on it, even if it was for fun."

Barnes assured Bavaro he wasn't going to get sick from *Fungi bartoli*. Bavaro looked over at McConkey, who burst out laughing. Bavaro opened the hotel window and tossed one of McConkey's possessions onto the street. He resisted any further revenge. "I was impressed by his sense of humor," Bavaro said. "That was a pretty good joke. Phil was eating it up. I was just so relieved I wasn't going to get sick. It showed what an idiot I am."

"I messed with him so badly," McConkey said.

No hard feelings?

"Not at all. We were all young and really just enjoyed playing," Bavaro said. "That '86 team was so unique. We were so tight. It was a credit to the environment Bill Parcells created and all the legendary players we had." Practical jokes are fun. Hazing and bullying are not. When it crosses the line, every player has a breaking point.

Carson was a sensational leader as the Giants made their run to the Super Bowl. Burt dumped the first bucket of Gatorade on Parcells following a victory in Washington in 1984, which has now become part of NFL tradition, but it was Carson who first turned it into a Giants tradition. Carson is a big man, a strong man, but a sensitive teddy bear with a huge heart. In the years before the 1986 season, though, it was not always easy for him to get along with everyone.

In particular, Banks was not feeling the love from Carson through training camp and early into his rookie season in 1984. He was the third overall pick at a position that was the strongest on a bad team. Carson and Taylor were the foundation of the defense with veterans Brad Van Pelt and Kelley. They were known as the "Crunch Bunch" and were close friends. When Taylor was drafted second overall in 1981, he was not immediately accepted by Carson, Van Pelt, and Kelley even though he was considered a generational talent. Two days before the draft, there was a newspaper report that the veterans on the team were threatening to boycott training camp to protest the contract they heard L.T. would be getting. Taylor was so unhappy he wrote a telegram to Giants coach Ray Perkins pleading with him not to draft him.

They didn't listen, of course. The Giants were a dreadful team, and management dared the vets not to show up. The Giants were bad with Carson, Kelley, and Van Pelt; they could be bad without them. The players all showed up, of course, and when at the first practice it became clear that Taylor was a freak of nature, they immediately accepted him, and the Giants made the playoffs in Taylor's first season for the first time since 1963.

Then the 1982 strike happened, and Perkins left at the end of the season to succeed his mentor and idol, Bear Bryant, at Alabama. Parcells was on the hot seat after his first season as the Giants head coach, and he knew changes needed to be made. Parcells wanted to get rid of Van Pelt and Kelley, who had experienced so much losing in their long careers in New York; he didn't want them spreading negative vibes to the younger players he planned to build around. Kelley was traded to the San Diego Chargers, Banks was drafted with the third overall pick in the 1984 draft, and then Van Pelt was traded to the Vikings.

Banks and Carson had a rough first few months together. Carson's two best friends were gone. Banks was even-keeled in the locker room, but he was also nobody's fool, and one day Carson pushed his hazing too far, which came close to starting a brawl in the shower. Instead, it was the turning point in a relationship that is still strong four decades later.

"Some of my friendships were forged literally through fire," Banks said. "I won't say I was welcomed with open arms as a linebacker because they had a very close-knit group with Brian, Brad, Harry, and Lawrence and with the guys under them too, with Andy Headen, Robbie Jones, and Byron Hunt. They were all very close. But that core four was really respected."

When Banks showed up at Pace University for his rookie training camp, Taylor and Carson were sitting outside the training room.

"I introduced myself, and Lawrence looks at me and says nothing," Banks said. "And Harry looks at me and says, 'So what the hell are you going to do to get on the field?' That was just kind of the beginning. As camp went on, this is a time when hazing would be pretty severe. I was hazed every day. Some of it was good natured, some of it was totally nefarious.

"Just, you know, name-calling. And there were only certain tasks that I would do, right? Just stuff. A lot of button pushing. You got to stand up and sing at lunch or breakfast or on demand, which was all fine, I could do that. But then they started giving me nicknames, and all kinds of stuff. You know, there's Jim Burt. A few other guys. And then there was Harry, who was the elder statesman but was the guy who was pushing the buttons a lot with me. Not so much Lawrence. So, it became kind of a daily ritual through training camp, and then even into the season, and I was just kind of not built to be bullied. It was good natured until it wasn't."

Carson said Banks's nickname was Chudd, which came from the movie *C.H.U.D.* (cannibalistic humanoid underground dwellers) a science-fiction movie that came out during Banks's rookie training camp. Call him Carl. Or Banks. Or Banksie. But not Chudd. Definitely not Chudd.

Banks played at 6'4", 235. Carson played at 6'2", 237.

Early in the 1984 season, Banks had enough of Carson.

After practice, they were taking showers. It was an open shower room like most locker rooms. No private stalls. Carson just wouldn't let up. "He thought it was okay to keep ragging on me," Banks said. "There's guys in the shower, and he thought it was funny and I didn't."

Carson was pushing the wrong buttons on the wrong person at the wrong time.

"I just snapped and was ready to fight," Banks said. "Stark naked in the shower."

Banks looked over at Carson with bad intentions. He didn't care who Harry Carson was. He was ready to knock him out.

"You keep talking, I'm going to whup your fucking ass," Banks said.

"You know I was just kidding, right?" Carson said.

"Shit's not funny anymore," Banks said.

There on the slippery shower floor, a serious injury was possible if a fight were to happen. The headlines in the New York tabloids would have been award winning. Fortunately, it didn't progress to the point that naked bodies were flying around. Carson backed off.

At first, Carson didn't recall the shower incident. Then, he said, "It wasn't anything major."

Banks had a different recollection.

"We're both standing there naked but I'm clearly ready to fight," Banks said. "He was like, 'Whoa, whoa, whoa, homeboy, I was just playing.' We talked after we got out of the shower. I told him I was sick of it and that was the end of it. We had a pretty big rookie class but I was the targeted one. Lawrence really didn't say a whole lot. He didn't haze. He was fun about it. To Harry, it was a little more personal. At the end of the day, you just have to prove your worth as a football player. With Harry, it was probably the thing that brought us closer together as teammates and friends, just him knowing what my boundaries were and me being willing to set them no matter what your status is as a captain or elder statesman."

Carson figured he was just putting Banks through what he considered normal rookie orientation. "We had nicknames for everybody," Carson said. His buddies Van Pelt and Kelley were pushed out, in Van Pelt's case because Banks played his position at outside linebacker opposite Taylor, and Carson missed them. Banks was a far superior player to either Van Pelt or Kelley, but when a fraternity has two of its brothers' memberships revoked, there are repercussions and innocent bystanders. Banks was caught in the crossfire.

"I didn't know anything about Carl except he went to Michigan State, which to me wasn't overwhelming with talent," Carson said. "As one of the veterans, we messed with everybody. By messing with everybody, you became part of the group, part of the team. I remember we wanted to see how good he can be and why you are a first-round pick."

Following the shower incident, Carson's hazing of Banks stopped. Nothing more from Carson or anybody else. Banks, Carson, and L.T., along with Gary Reasons, another rookie in 1984, comprised the '86 Giants best unit and made so many big plays to lead them to the Super Bowl. "Harry and I to this day are as close as can be," Banks said.

If a player can dish it out, he'd also better be able to take it. If a player has a quirk, other players will pick up on it in a minute. Thin skin not allowed.

Not surprisingly, sex was a constant topic. One day Burt noticed a totally naked player admiring himself in front of a mirror off to the side of the weight room. He gathered teammates to check out the show and give him shit. One player bragged that he ran out of the locker room after his morning meeting and had sex with multiple women before returning for the afternoon practice. That same player used to walk around the locker room with a cutoff T-shirt and nothing else. "Disgusting," Burt said.

When the Giants get together for reunions, the locker room hierarchy of 1986 is restored. The needlers still needle. The picked on still get picked on.

"One of the fun times was always sitting at your locker and having fifteen or twenty minutes before we had to be on the field, and just listening to everybody," Simms said. "Some things that were said, you laugh until you cry. It was hilarious. The linemen had all kinds of personalities, and they would be instigators. But the whole group would get involved. It was a great mixture, socially, racially, and economically. I can remember it like it was yesterday."

Simms could tease. And he could take it. He endeared himself to his linemen when he became one of the first quarterbacks to make sure the five guys starting up front became his buddies. He would come in early to lift weights with them or would stay late to lift with them.

Then he would sit around his locker to shoot the shit, and they would make fun of one another.

The Giants training facilities during the season in the stadium were spartan. The weight room was in a dimly lit area off the locker room. In their current training headquarters, the weight room looks like a health club. There was no cafeteria with a menu designed by nutritionists providing breakfast and lunch as there is today. When Simms left his house in the morning, his wife Diana packed him lunch with a sandwich, an apple, and a cupcake. "I felt like I was going to school," he said. Every Friday, Simms ordered pizza to be delivered to the locker room for the entire team after practice. He wasn't trying to buy anybody's friendship, but sitting around eating pizza after a long week of practice brought the team even closer together.

Taylor could be a jokester, but players were wary about sending any verbal zingers his way for fear of physical retaliation.

"Lawrence is not only scary and intimidating but he's one of the funniest guys I've ever seen," Mark Bavaro said.

Parcells was almost completely off limits, except for Taylor.

Parcells was never put off when a player talked back. The practice field at camp at Pace University didn't drain well. When the field was soaked, the players had to walk through a path in the woods to practice at Briarcliff High School, which was on higher ground. On the way back through the woods, Parcells was teasing Taylor about a play he messed up in practice.

"Parcells is clowning L.T.," Pepper Johnson said.

He said Taylor and Carson could "buddy-buddy talk" with Parcells and get away with just about anything. But Taylor never wanted to be embarrassed in front of his teammates, even when he knew Parcells was kidding. The players wanting to kiss Parcells's ass laughed as he kept going after Taylor. That encouraged Parcells to keep piling on. "So, Parcells got a little air in his chest," Johnson said. "He was poking the bear."

L.T. was getting increasingly pissed off with each insult. Parcells told Taylor he wasn't scared of him. "I know those guys have a close relationship, but I was thinking if that was me, man, I got to shut this dude up," Johnson said.

Parcells grabbed Taylor. "You don't want none of this," Taylor said.

L.T. struggled to get free of Parcells's grip, and everybody was laughing at him. That soon changed. As soon as they cleared the woods, "L.T. this time attacks Parcells. He grabs him and lifts him up over his head," Johnson said. "L.T. didn't want to flip him and take him to the ground."

He carried his coach over to a parking lot. "He dropped him on top of the roof of a car," Johnson said.

"I remember that," Parcells laughed.

Now the players who were laughing at Taylor were laughing at Parcells. "I told you to quit playing," Taylor said.

Parcells had that "red-in-the-face smile," Johnson said.

The players helped him down from the car. More than ten years later, when Parcells was coaching the Jets and Johnson was playing for them, Johnson said Parcells was telling his players how he stood up one day to Taylor at training camp. "Wait a minute," Johnson said to Parcells. "Do you want me to say the part about when he lifts you up and puts you on top of the car?"

Taylor is the best player Parcells ever coached. Parcells is the best coach Taylor had in his career. Their ability to tease each other created a playful spirit in the Giants locker room. If something went wrong on the field or Parcells got word there was division in the locker room, he relied on Carson and Martin to take care of it. After a dismal defensive showing in Dallas in the '86 season-opening loss, Parcells and Carson decided a players-only dinner was necessary to get the team back on track. Parcells turned over the fine money to Carson that he had collected throughout training camp for various rules violations to pay the bill, which came to $150–$200 a man times forty-five.

They did not eat at pricey Ruth's Chris or Morton's. It was a blue-collar dinner for a blue-collar team at Beefsteak Charlie's on Route 17 in New Jersey. Carson declared attendance was mandatory, and offense, defense, special teams, and even Taylor showed up. "We eat like animals and drink like fish," Leonard Marshall said. "And Harry would pay the bill."

It was another piece to the puzzle of the Giants becoming a brotherhood. Carson called dinner meetings three or four times a year. "I think those dinners had a lot to do with the unity, the camaraderie, the building of a fraternity," Marshall said. "And you saw it evidenced in the way we played. We congratulated each other, we celebrated each other. The cohesiveness and the effort that we gave to each other was amazing."

The dinners helped players get to know each other. If any Black or white cliques were developing, the dinners dissolved them. Marshall, a Black man from Franklin, Louisiana, said he wanted to get to know everything about Billy Ard, a white guard from East Orange, New Jersey.

After the loss to Dallas, in a typical Parcells rant, he called the media "commies." He always said it with a smile but also took measures to prevent the massive amount of press covering the Giants from splitting the team. After the Dallas loss, it was decided to boycott the media.

"Who was the ringleader?" Marshall said. "Fucking Harry."

There was a television room right off the entrance to the locker room. At first, Marshall said only Black players would congregate. "The next thing you know some of the white players are coming to the room," he said. "You know what? This is cool. You guys should be in this fucking room. Come in here, hang out and bullshit with us."

The locker room is the melting pot of sports. Players from all areas of the country need to come together as one despite being of different racial, ethnic, religious, political, and financial backgrounds. "It is so interesting to be a part of guys who went to different schools, different backgrounds, different races, different social classes, different religions—you are all thrown together," Carson said. "And you are working for that one goal and that is to win. You don't see color, you don't see political affiliations, you don't see anything except that guy next to you is your brother."

Complete harmony, however, is not realistic, especially during a period of racial tension in New York. Giants players, Black and white, insist Parcells constructed a locker room that kept conflict to a minimum. Linebacker Pepper Johnson was told by one of his friends on the team in 1988 that a white teammate from the South called him a "cocky n-word." Johnson said he confronted the player, who apologized and invited him to dinner at his house to smooth things over. Johnson felt because the teammate had never invited him to dinner before this incident, he wasn't about to go over now. So he declined.

Black and white players insist it was a prejudice-free locker room and the situation with Johnson was a one-off. Martin made sure of it. "We confirmed it, we addressed it. And we got support from the coaches, because that was not to be tolerated," Martin said. "So, we didn't sweep it under the rug, didn't act like it didn't happen. And then you put it behind you, and you try to go forward. Of course, you never forget it, but you don't allow it to be an impediment to success."

Collins, who had played high school and college football in California, appreciated the predominantly color-free approach of his teammates.

"Once we got into the locker room, there was nothing. We were Giants. I didn't see any racial hatred," Collins said. "We went out to dinner as a team in '86 more than any other team I played on, and I played thirteen years."

"I don't think we ever thought about the racial part," Maurice Carthon said.

Parcells spent most of his Hall of Fame speech talking about the dynamics of the locker room and how he tried to build a talented team with the right chemistry. Bavaro thinks the culture of the team led to the Super Bowl title, rather than the other way around. "He collected personalities as much as talent," Bavaro said. "There were certain types of players who wouldn't cut it in the Giants locker room. On other teams I was on, talent seemed to rule the day, regardless of however everyone got along. Chemistry was one of the Giants' biggest weapons."

When a team is run by Parcells, a no-nonsense coach, and his consigliere is Belichick, nicknamed "Doom" for always expecting the worst, it was incumbent upon the players to find some humor to keep from bouncing off the walls of the locker room.

On the last day of training camp at Pace, the Giants couldn't wait to get out of the dorms, where the beds were too small and the mattresses too thin, and race south on the Saw Mill River Parkway, presuming heavy rains had not turned it into the Saw Mill Riverway, and get back to the comfort of their homes and apartments in New Jersey. "We stayed in a girls' dorm at Pace with tiny beds," Simms said. "I would lie in bed at night and think, 'What am I doing in this room? Why can't I drive home at night?'"

Simms missed the amenities of home, especially the comfort of knowing he wasn't going to be pranked in his own bedroom.

Jim Burt was the Giants' number-one class clown. He was from the University of Miami, signed by the Giants as an undrafted free agent in 1981. He became one of the best nose tackles in the NFL, benefiting from the coaching of Parcells and Belichick, as well as Carson playing directly behind him in the Giants 3-4 alignment. As camp was closing, Burt plotted to take care of his pal Simms. "He had a new Mercedes, we stole the keys and parked it on the other side of campus," Burt said. "It was the last day of training camp, so everyone was itching to get out of there."

Before Simms could realize his $50,000 car was missing, Burt had another trick planned to start the day. He grabbed a fire extinguisher off the wall and pulled the trigger and shot it under Simms's door. "I thought it was just water," Burt said. "But it shoots this white foam. I didn't know that. I stick it underneath his door and I let it loose. Simms was sleeping and he yells out like he's getting killed. Holy shit. He scared the shit out of me. I ran my ass off I was so scared."

The good news for Simms is that Burt didn't empty the fire extinguisher in his new car. Burt might have landed the first shot, but Simms was his equal as a practical joker. Burt knew he was going to retaliate—he just had no idea when or how. One of the proven winners was to load up a teammate's shorts with a generous amount of pain relief ointment that burns when it interacts with perspiration.

"It's a paste," Burt said. "And then you let it sit there overnight."

He would know. It's how Simms got his revenge. The rest of the team knew Burt's thighs and private area were about to feel like a five-alarm fire. After a few reps in practice, all eyes were on Burt.

"You put it in there overnight and then you don't smell it, but then as soon as you start sweating, your balls are on fire," Burt said. "I realized everybody was watching. I didn't say a word. Then I ran in and changed my shorts. They got me good but I didn't let them know. Every day was something different."

Defensive line coach Lamar Leachman was from Cartersville, Georgia, spoke with a thick accent, and loved to yell at his players. He also liked all things free, even if they weren't necessarily free. Such as raiding the hotel housekeeper's cart of towels, soap, and shampoo. "He was a kleptomaniac," Burt said. "He would steal everything from everyone."

A group of players were on to him and waited around the corner in the hallway for Leachman to pilfer the cart.

"Hey!" they yelled at Leachman.

He was startled.

"He jumped out of his ass and says, 'You got me, boys, you got me,'" Burt said.

Leachman was well known for hoarding his per diem on road trips and using the money to buy his wife Christmas presents. On road trips, the Giants would have a "5 o'clock club" for the coaches and media in the team hotel. Leachman would load up on appetizers and pocket his dinner money. He would walk around the locker room late in the season reminding players that playoff money was at stake. At the beginning of minicamp in the spring, the coaches were issued a set of brand-new Giants shorts and T-shirts. After the other coaches threw their dirty clothes in the laundry at the end of practice, Leachman all but dove into the basket to retrieve the clothes and then was courteous enough to wash them. Why? A few nights later a bunch of the coaches went over to Manny's, a restaurant-bar in Moonachie, ten minutes from the stadium. It was owned by Manny Cimiluca, a devoted Giants fan, who was tight with Parcells and Ed Croke. It was the go-to place for the coaches, with lots of Giants fans.

When Parcells, Belichick, and some of the other coaches came by a few hours after work, they noticed the bartenders, waiters, and waitresses decked out in brand-new Giants shirts, which happened to belong to the coaches.

In return for free food and drinks, Leachman delivered the Giants gear to Manny's.

"Belichick is such a ballbuster and you can't put anything past him," Burt said.

"Hey, that looks like my freaking shirt," Belichick said. "Where did you get those shirts?"

"Oh, from Lamar. He is such a nice guy. He came with the shirts," one of the members of Manny's staff said.

"He stole them from us the first day of minicamp," Belichick said.

Assistant coaches rarely made over $125,000 in the '80s, but that was likely still enough for Leachman to buy his own dinner at Manny's. "He just wanted free shit," Burt said. "He traded them for drinks and told them, 'I got more stuff. Don't worry about it.'"

Strength coach Johnny Parker was known for being cheap and a scavenger like Leachman but, more important, for his penchant for wanting his name in the newspaper. So, Burt and others hired a stripper, told Parker a female reporter from the *New York Daily News* wanted to interview him for a big story, and conspired with the team's public relations department to bring her into the weight room area near the locker room to do the interview. Parker didn't flinch as Burt blasted striptease music on the locker room speakers and the woman first opened and then removed her shirt at Parker's eye level in a memorable fifteen-minute performance. "We laughed our ass off," Burt said.

In keeping with the change in locker room culture since 1986 to a more politically correct environment, bringing in a stripper to dance in front of an assistant coach would surely result in a big fine and suspension, if not the player getting placed on waivers. In 1986, they all just laughed.

The players saved the best payback for Leachman, who also made a habit out of stealing chewing tobacco out of Benson's locker. Benson had an endorsement deal and was a generous guy, allowing others to share in the dip. During the season, the tobacco cans were lined up in his locker, and Leachman freely borrowed without asking, much like he did with the hotel shampoo. The locker space at training camp, however, was tiny, leaving Benson room to store only one can. The players hated the practice field and not just because it didn't drain well. Geese were prevalent in the area, and every morning goose droppings littered the field sideline to sideline, end zone to end zone. Usually a team's pre-practice stretching line is straight as a ruler, but the Giants' was as crooked as a drunkard's walk. It zigzagged as players searched for a spot to lay their head without coming to rest in a pile of goose shit.

Benson and Burt decided it was time to teach Leachman a tasty lesson about dipping into the dip without asking. "He was pissing off Brad," Burt said. "Brad was missing Copenhagen just nonstop."

"What to do?" Benson asked.

"Put goose shit in there," Burt suggested.

"You go get it," Benson said.

"I would love to but keep me out of this. He's my position coach," Burt said.

Burt went out to the practice field and scooped up some goose poop and left the rest of the prank to Benson. He handed the poopy tissue to Benson, who mixed it into the dip with his fingers. He placed the can of Copenhagen on the shelf in his locker, knowing it would attract Leachman like a bee to honey. Leachman arrived at practice while the players were stretching.

He walked through the stretching lines with Benson's Copenhagen tucked in its customary visible spot in his sock. Benson and Burt filled in ten other players on what was about to go down. Leachman removed the can from his sock and put in a pinch between his cheek and gum. Burt was laughing so hard he could have peed in his pants.

Ten seconds go by. Then it happened.

"Benson, boy, this Copenhagen *tastes like shit!*" Leachman barked. Burt couldn't help himself.

"Because it is shit!" he responded.

Leachman spit up and ran into the locker room to rinse out his mouth and clean his hands. "It was the best comeback ever," Burt said.

Silly stuff, for sure, but all part of the behind-the-scenes interactions that bonded the '86 Giants and inspired them to play hard for each other. Even play hard for Leachman. They didn't mess with Parcells. He was the boss. They didn't mess with Belichick. He was all business. They didn't mess with L.T. They were scared of him. But Phil Simms, the quarterback who would go on to perform at the highest level in the Super Bowl, was right in the middle of the nonsense, and that made just about everybody else fair game to be picked on.

By 1986, there was no hazing of rookies. Once on the team, the locker room became the sanctuary for every player, regardless of status. "I think people play their best when they play for each other," Bavaro said.

The '86 Giants grew closer by having fun with one another. And as the games went on, winning made the brotherhood even tighter. Still, when the lights were turned off, the cheering stopped, and they walked out of the stadium for the very last time, grabbing their jersey and helmet as a keepsake, they were as vulnerable to the pitfalls of life as anybody else.

2

DARK DAYS

**Mark Bavaro's living room,
Boxford, Massachusetts, February 2022**

Mark Bavaro's house on a quiet street with picturesque property twenty-five miles north of Boston and twenty-three miles south of the New Hampshire border is the epitome of New England charm. He has a room with football memorabilia, but it is understated, fitting his personality, and really nothing about him is a dead giveaway that he's a two-time Super Bowl champion and an ultraphysical player who was the best tight end in New York Giants history.

Except the rows of prescription bottles on the island in his kitchen.

"Look in here," he said, opening a kitchen cabinet.

Just as many bottles. This was the first group of the pills he no longer needs. Altogether between the island and the cabinet, there are enough pills to take care of an entire football team and practice squad.

They are all for him.

Bavaro suffered from a debilitating case of long-term Covid, and until doctors finally found the right cocktail of pills to settle him down, his anxiety, paranoia, dizziness, fogginess, and headaches had him believing life was no longer worth living. It had him sitting up at night contemplating suicide.

"You think about it," he said. "You're like, 'What the fuck?' You're on top of a burning building and how long can you stay there until you jump off? You come to understand a lot about other people and what they go through."

This seemingly indestructible former All-Pro who symbolized the heart of blue-collar New Yorkers in his playing days, who ran over and dragged half the 49ers defense in an inspiring run-after-the-catch at Candlestick Park in 1986, was overwhelmed by a disease that was new even to the pain-wracked fraternity of former football players. Death, he debated in his darkest time, had to be better than the nonstop turmoil raging in his brain that had been attacked by Covid. And he had to wonder whether he had been made more vulnerable by all the hits to the head he sustained playing football. He won't blame football but won't rule it out.

Bavaro went to Notre Dame with safety Dave Duerson, and they later played together on the Giants 1990 Super Bowl championship team. He played one season with hard-hitting safety Andre "Dirty" Waters in Philadelphia at the end of his career. He never played with Hall of Fame linebacker Junior Seau, but they became friends through defensive end Burt Grossman, a teammate of Seau's in San Diego.

Duerson, Waters, and Seau all were diagnosed with CTE. The diagnosis can only be made posthumously. They all died by suicide, and their families donated their brains for CTE research and evaluation. And it wasn't just his NFL colleagues. A couple of Bavaro's friends he went to school with at Danvers High School in Massachusetts killed themselves. A friend's mother died by suicide. Bavaro couldn't quite make sense of it. Could life be so bad that you make the choice to leave behind wives, children, grandchildren, parents, and friends? Wasn't it the coward's way out? Didn't only selfish people check out and take their own life?

In the depths of his battle with Covid, he started to think about it. Bavaro never planned how to end his life, but "you think of ways. How does one die?" he said. "I was praying for a heart attack."

Even with an ablation procedure in 2015 to treat atrial fibrillation, Bavaro's heart was beating strong. It meant he would have to consciously decide to leave his wife Susan and his adult children. The debate kept raging inside him. The pain wasn't football pain. He long ago became conditioned to feeling like crap on Monday mornings and just about every morning during his playing years. It was his emotional side that was damaged, insisting life really sucked with no end to his misery in sight. "I had to stick to my intellectual side and say, 'Your life is good,'" he said. "Before I got sick, I was happy as a clam playing golf and hanging out. I was not making a ton of money but was making enough to get by. The kids were great, the wife's great, everything was great. There was nothing to be depressed about."

His mind was playing tricks. Should he listen to his emotional side, the dangerous side? Or the intellectual side, the rational side? He wanted to believe the intellectual side, but the emotional side was presenting a strong argument. The intellectual side had lost its credibility. "Things were so bad that I wished I was dead," he said. "I wished that somehow, I would just die. Once you get to that point . . ."

The antidepressants magnified his suicidal thoughts, which he learned could be a side effect, and a side effect of Covid as well. He sat up nights in his living room chair trying to convince himself that life was indeed good and the train would soon get back on the tracks. "It's not like I looked at my life and was saying what's the point or there's no hope for my life," he said. "My body and mind were out of whack. It wasn't pain in the traditional sense. It was feelings and sensations that were unbearable. I had to put aside my feelings side because they were in some other place that I didn't understand."

He came to understand how Duerson, Waters, and Seau pulled the trigger, but Bavaro's intellectual side fortunately won out. He didn't point a gun at himself or line up a lethal combination of pills or drink himself to death or go out on the streets of Boston and buy a lethal amount of crack to smoke. Even if he hated the nickname teammates gave him as a rookie in 1985, he was still the person who'd earned it: Rambo. Bavaro was a tough guy, and he would not give in.

Bavaro's inner strength was being tested, for sure. He slowly started to feel more like himself by the summer of 2022 and was able to return to the golf course on a semi-regular basis. He is passionate about golf. But even that turned into another challenge by late August. After his tee shot landed in the rough, he surveyed the lie but could not determine exactly what was under the ball. Was it grass? Shrubs? Branches? Rocks? He didn't move the ball to find out but also knew he had to be careful. He took a half swing to get back onto the fairway, but a rock jumped up and hit him so fast he was not able to close his eye. The rock hit him flush in the eye and scratched his retina, and he was back in the emergency room with lightning bolt flashes interfering with his vision.

By that point, it was just piling on.

====

MARK BAVARO WAS sitting by his locker at his first minicamp in 1985. The rookies came in ahead of the veterans, a group of whom the night before reporting had been to the movies to see *Rambo*, a movie starring Sylvester Stallone about a Vietnam War veteran returning home.

"Hey, there's Rambo," one of the Giants veteran players said, pointing at Bavaro.

Bavaro looked like Stallone. He had the same long hair. Even mumbled like Rocky. But since his new teammates had not seen him on the field yet, *Rambo* was not a nod to him being a tough army guy. It was more about his looks.

But once Bavaro started running over defenders in games, it stuck for good. "He is tough," they said, "like Rambo."

Mark's uncle Donald Bavaro and his cousin Bobby Rossi were Vietnam vets, and Bavaro thought the nickname was disrespectful to those who served in the war. "Not to be self-righteous or anything, but I really thought and still do that it was an honor to serve there, as shitty as it was. Donald managed to transition back into civilian life, but Bobby came home from Vietnam and had a bunch of drug problems," Bavaro said. "I think it aged him."

Bobby became a recluse in Florida when he returned from Vietnam. He died in his sixties. Bavaro doesn't know the circumstances of his cousin's death. Bobby didn't even attend his own father's funeral, although he later visited his family privately. Bavaro sees his uncle Donald often. Because he had family fighting in Vietnam, he would have been happy with just about any other nickname. "I just didn't like it," he said. "Rocky, I would have been fine with. If Rambo wasn't a Vietnam vet, I would have been yeah, yeah, great. Whatever you want. I wish they would have just called me Mark."

Still, Bavaro's toughness was legendary.

At the end of a 1986 game against the Cardinals, he was upset with Simms for taking a knee in victory formation with the outcome decided. According to what players told Parcells, Niko Noga, a linebacker for the Cardinals, had spit in Bavaro's face early in the game, and Bavaro took every opportunity to hit Noga with clean shots the rest of the way.

"Six tight diamond, kill the clock," Simms shouted in the huddle, giving his teammates the signal that they were going to kneel out the rest of the game.

Bavaro made a disapproving noise and gave Simms the death stare.

"What's the matter with you?" Simms asked.

"I want to hit that motherfucker once more," Bavaro said.

Simms took the knee.

Early in the first quarter of another 1986 game, he took a short pass from Simms, broke a tackle by Saints safety Frank Wattelet and ran upfield before he was brought down and injured by a helmet-to-facemask hit by cornerback Antonio Gibson, with Wattelet falling on top of him. Bavaro suffered what was initially reported to the media during the game as a chipped tooth.

Turned out he had a broken jaw.

"I'm telling you, I'm looking at him, and there's blood gushing under his teeth," Parcells said. "And they put on this stuff where they can just throw it in your mouth and it stops the bleeding. They get that done. [Team dentist] Dr. [Hugh] Gardi does that. And then they take him in the dressing room, because they're going to x-ray him."

The x-ray room was in the corridor down the hall from the Giants locker room in the bowels of the stadium. "I remember them saying it looked fractured but that the x-ray machine in the tunnel was not high quality," Bavaro said. "So, they weren't sure how bad it was, if it was broken. I knew something was wrong because I could feel my teeth moving and there was nothing wrong with them. It was the bone moving. That's why there were initial reports that I had some teeth knocked out. There was a lot of blood, too, but I'm not sure from where, which added to the story. They suspected a broken jaw but couldn't say definitively, otherwise they probably wouldn't have let me return to the game."

The Giants were down 17–3 when Bavaro came back out of the tunnel late in the second quarter. "So the game is going on," Parcells said. "And all of a sudden, Bavaro hits me in the back." Parcells imitates a grunting sound he said Bavaro was making. "That means, 'I'm ready to go,'" Parcells said. "He catches a touchdown pass. He was something. I loved him."

Bavaro would catch a 24-yard pass to set up his 19-yard touchdown from Simms before halftime, inspiring a 20–17 victory. He finished with seven catches for 110 yards.

Why would he come back in the game after breaking his jaw?

"Because I could," he said. "There was not much you can do about it. Play or don't play. I felt I could still play and so I did willingly. If I didn't feel I could've played, I certainly wouldn't have, and they wouldn't have forced me to, either. It all happened pretty fast, and as you know, there's a degree of chaos, confusion, and multiple problems during a game. My injury wasn't a huge priority. More like 'we'll figure it out later.' I've had other injuries where I couldn't play.

Little things like my [broken] toe. I could play with a broken jaw or my shoulder out of joint or my knee falling apart. It was just the things I could bear, you know? The things I couldn't, I didn't."

The Giants were not a team that believed in painkiller injections to get or keep players on the field. "I asked for a shot once as a rookie for a sprained ankle. They just laughed at me," Bavaro said. "Cleveland, Philly [where he later played], different story. Either they had integrity or were inhumane. I like to think the Giants had integrity. Ronnie Barnes is a good man."

He went home that night and tried to eat. He needed something soft and easy to swallow. "I had French onion soup but couldn't eat the cheese," he said. "That was more painful than playing the rest of the game. Life is funny."

The next morning, he was in the dentist's chair having his jaw wired shut. It stayed that way for five weeks, but he kept playing. He brought a blender on the road and sipped eggplant parmigiana through a straw. There are many players who are warriors, play with pain, and sacrifice their bodies for the team. Bavaro was one of those guys. If knee injuries hadn't curtailed his career, he would have been on a Hall of Fame track. Post-career toward the end of 2018, he had knee and shoulder replacements three months apart, so common among former players.

=====

BAVARO'S HEALTH STRUGGLES go back to April 4, 2021. His daughter, her husband, and their baby came over to the house for an Easter Sunday visit. The next day, his daughter and her family were not feeling well and all tested positive for Covid. "I was holding the baby," Bavaro said. He had not yet been vaccinated and was in close contact. "No one else caught it from them. It was just me," he said.

He played golf the next two days after Easter and came home the second night feeling like he had a cold. "I knew I had it," he said. "I just assumed it was Covid."

That began an odyssey that inflicted more mental and physical pain than anything he experienced during his nine-year career in the

NFL. Susan, who now teaches Advanced Placement European history and constitutional law in high school, believes the problems caused by Covid trace to Bavaro's football days before the NFL adopted a concussion protocol with strict guidelines for when players were allowed to return to the field. Her research led her to conclude that viruses such as Covid attack the most vulnerable part of the body, which in Bavaro's case quite possibly was his brain, which had rattled inside his skull with each jarring hit. "I know my wife wants to make that claim and she may be right," Bavaro said. "I just don't want to come off that I'm laying the blame for my Covid woes on the NFL."

Week one after contracting Covid was bad. "It never went to my lungs. It went to my head," he said. "And my head was just swirling."

Week two was worse. He still felt like he had a cold. He was having trouble sleeping, so he stayed up, trying to get tired. It was just about bedtime. Susan was already asleep upstairs and Bavaro was in the kitchen of his four-bedroom house. He started to feel light-headed and found himself on the kitchen floor. He had passed out. "I had just enough strength to get to a chair by the island in the kitchen," he said.

"Susan!" he called out.

She ran down the steps and found her husband woozy. "The next thing I know she was by my side and on the phone," he said.

"What are you doing?" he asked.

"I'm calling 911," she said.

He knew once the call to 911 was placed, it would bring a parade of paramedics to his house. But he was Mark Bavaro, 6'4", 245 pounds, and strong as hell in his football days, and he didn't need help. He didn't want help. But he was no longer a twenty-three-year-old kid playing with a broken jaw. He was a fifty-eight-year-old middle-aged man who fainted on his kitchen floor. The paramedics checked his vitals, which were fine, and he avoided a trip to the emergency room. "They told me not to go to the hospital, that it would be more trouble than it's worth because there's nothing they can probably do for you," he said. "I said great. So, they left."

But it wasn't over. He developed insomnia, which went on for months. The day after passing out in the kitchen, he had a good day. He stayed up late again, way after Susan, knowing he was going to have a tough time falling asleep. He made it up the stairs to the bedroom without a problem and lay down in bed. That's when it hit him. "It was like a tornado going on in my head and I couldn't stand it," he said. "It was driving me crazy." He didn't want to wake up Susan, but he couldn't fall asleep. He got up to go to the bathroom two steps from his bed. "I felt this click and clench in my gut, my diaphragm, and it radiated up," he said.

He remembers thinking to himself, *Shit, I'm going to pass out again.*

Bavaro made it to the edge of his bed and sat down facing the bathroom door. Susan picked up her head. "You okay?" she asked.

He stood up to try to make it to the bathroom again. He passed out again and this time the fall was violent. He went down face first on the threshold to the bathroom. "The next thing you know, I was on the floor of the marble tile of my bathroom in a pool of blood," he said. "Blood was just pouring out of my nose."

Susan called 911 again. This time when the ambulance came, they took him to the ER. He was told in the ER that he was dehydrated. He was there for five hours, but he said it took three hours for them to administer fluid. He needed stitches to sew up the inside of his mouth. He had wrenched his neck. He had unforgiving headaches. "That was the beginning of all my troubles," he said. "There were months, *months*, where I just wanted to die. I really did."

As he was telling me this story, he said, "Come look at this."

He took out his cell phone and scrolled to pictures from April 2021. He found one taken in the hospital after the bathroom fall. He had black eyes that stretched from one side of each eye to the bridge of his nose. His face was bruised. He looked like he went twelve rounds with Muhammad Ali . . .with his hands tied behind his back.

"I really ripped my nose up. I think I had a concussion. And my neck was off," he said. "The hat trick, you know. I had three things going on. I was a wreck. I was a mess."

At least he didn't break his nose. That surprised him. "Lots of stitches and lots of divots in what used to be a pretty smooth nose," he said. "I can still feel the blow almost two years later. I don't know the exact cause of the black and blue. No one seemed too interested in it."

One of Bavaro's business associates who deals with his memorabilia told him she had Covid and it went to her lungs. One night she, too, fainted in her bathroom and hit her face on the bathtub. They exchanged pictures of their injuries. "We were like, oh my God, we're twins," he said. "It was almost the exact same injury. So, it's not unique to me. There were a lot of other people who were going through this. I don't know what their neurological situation was prior. But they can't all have been football players or involved in head trauma. I think it's just a symptom of the virus."

All those years in the NFL going against strongside linebackers and strong safeties and absorbing defenseless blindside hits and helmet-to-helmet blows—and fainting face first on the bathroom floor did the most damage. It confused him how he did so much harm to himself when he had survived such a physical sport. He discussed it with a psychiatrist he had grown to trust. Unfortunately, she didn't take his insurance, and the out-of-pocket expense became overwhelming. He had no choice but to change doctors.

Bavaro received the Covid vaccine two months after he was infected. He considered getting the shot before he got Covid but had not made up his mind, and, besides, it was not yet readily available for his age group. For months after the fall in the bathroom, he had a swollen feeling in his sinuses, his head felt full, and every time he told friends he was turning the corner, things instead turned bad again. He was stuck in a vicious cycle. "My head was bursting at the seams," he said. "It felt like my brain was boiling. I couldn't move. I had fatigue. The noise in my head was just unrelenting."

At least he had Susan to care for him. Bavaro couldn't even get out of bed, but then she got Covid and was sick for ten days. His sons came from New York and stayed in the house in Boxford for two weeks taking care of them. "We were both in bed," Bavaro said. "It was like *Willy Wonka*, you know, the family that stayed in bed."

Once Susan recovered, she began taking Bavaro to doctors. A lot of doctors. The NFL Players Association negotiated a new plan for health care in the collective bargaining agreement in 2020 that helped with Bavaro's medical expenses. He started to feel a little better by August 2021 and decided to participate in a card-signing show in Poughkeepsie, New York, with former teammates Lawrence Taylor, Joe Morris, and Rodney Hampton. "Halfway through, I almost passed out again," he said. "I had to leave. It was embarrassing."

New York Giants Training Camp, 1985, Pace University, Pleasantville, New York

Still, the card signing was about memories and friendships. And those things—along with the money, of course—are what makes playing a physically demanding game worth it. Bavaro played in the NFL for three teams and left with two Super Bowl championships and a spot in the Giants Ring of Honor. He had an eventful journey starting with his rookie training camp in 1985.

Bavaro was a fourth-round draft choice from Notre Dame looking forward to his only night off after a tough first week of practice. Summer camp was a grind back in the '80s when it lasted six weeks, and Parcells loved to run two-a-days in pads day after day in oppressive 85-degree heat to separate the ballers from the boys who drop like a shanked punt.

One week can feel like three, which is why players cherish their one free night each week. Bavaro was ready for a break after reporting early with his rookie class and then going up against the strong group of veteran Giants linebackers. He needed to chill out and let it rip.

He brought with him from college a fondness for drinking.

Whiskey.

A lot of whiskey.

After the second grueling practice leading up to their free night, the Giants had a team-building barbeque on campus for players and coaches, and then the players were on their own until the 11 p.m. curfew. Manhattan was thirty miles away, too far with few precious hours available, so Bavaro stayed local, which presumably gave him a better chance to make curfew. He was physically imposing and would soon prove he could catch, run, and block with the best, but with the tight-end room composed of holdovers Zeke Mowatt, Don Hasselbeck, and Gary Shirk, just making the team was his goal. Bill Parcells didn't pass out compliments to a rookie so early in camp, which led to insecurity, even though the Giants were not good enough to cut a relatively high draft pick.

"I never knew where I stood," Bavaro said.

Nine months earlier, he was having lunch with his Notre Dame teammates in the Giants Stadium press box the day before a November game against Navy that the Irish would win on a last-second field goal. The Giants were leaving for a trip to Dallas the next day, and Bavaro looked wide eyed as the team paraded onto the field for their Friday afternoon walk-through. Bavaro was from the Boston area but wasn't a huge football fan—former Irish tight end Dave Casper was his favorite player—and looked in awe at the size of NFL players.

"Oh, that's Lawrence Taylor. That's Carl Banks and Harry Carson. That's Andy Headen and Byron Hunt," one of his teammates pointed out.

"What are they? Defensive linemen?" Bavaro asked.

"No, those are linebackers," he was told.

Oh shit.

Bavaro was now going head to head in practice with L.T., Banks, and Carson, trying to bury them on sweeps by Joe Morris and get a step on them to catch passes over the middle from Phil Simms. He was no longer in South Bend facing undersized linebackers and slow safeties he could dominate. Taylor was on his way to being the best defensive player in NFL history, Carson was a future Hall of Famer as well, and Banks would surely be in Canton, too, if he hadn't been overshadowed by Taylor. Every play, every practice, was a battle for Bavaro. At least he received some much-needed positive reinforcement a couple of weeks into camp.

"I ran a seam pattern down the middle. Phil Simms threw it, and I made a nice catch in the end zone, and I jogged back to the huddle," he said. "And Parcells came up to me and said, 'Good play, kid. You looked good doing it.' He patted me on the ass. That's the first indication I had that I think I'm doing okay."

Bavaro hit his first night off like a lion sprung from the Bronx Zoo. He'd survived week one and wanted to celebrate with drinks. There was still a long way to go to make the roster, but he knew he couldn't pace himself in practice. Parcells's calendar had no load management days. Bavaro needed to make an impression to move up the depth chart and force his way on the field. He must have forgotten he needed to pace himself with his drinking. He was known by teammates and coaches throughout his career as a quiet guy, very difficult to read, but his behavior that first night out was quite the opposite.

Bavaro lined his stomach with burgers and a couple of beers at the team picnic, then hit the streets of picturesque Pleasantville. His objective was simply to have some farewell fun with camp roommate "Touchdown" Tony Baker, a rookie free agent running back from Cornell, who knew he was being released the next morning. Bavaro's group stopped off at one pub before descending on Michael's, a sports bar on Bedford Road just a couple of miles from the Pace campus. The bartender poured Bavaro a glass of whiskey. Then another. "I don't know how much I drank, but I was drunk," he said.

Running back John Tuggle showed up. He was diagnosed with cancer in 1984, tried to make a comeback in minicamp in 1985, but wasn't cleared to participate in training camp. The Giants allowed him to remain on the roster so his medical bills would be paid. Tuggle passed away the next year. "I didn't really know him, but he was nice to me," Bavaro said. "I kind of knew his story. He starts doing shots of tequila and is bringing the young guys up to the bar. I was like, 'Wow, this was a veteran wanting to drink with us. That's pretty cool.'"

Bavaro remained at Michael's way too long and lost track of time until he looked at his watch. It was 2 a.m. "Shit, I missed curfew," he said. "I missed bed check."

═══

IT WAS NOT just lateness. He's not sure why, but he started punching walls in Michael's. And when a bar patron said something to aggravate him, his reaction was way over the top. "I grabbed some guy and threw him over the bar," he said.

Not good.

"It wasn't in a violent way," he said, laughing. "I wasn't punching anybody. I was *fucking* drunk. I was so drunk."

The manager at Michael's made it clear he was no longer welcome at his establishment. He was banned for life. Bavaro managed to get back to the dorms and didn't care that the thin mattresses were made for college kids and not professional football players. He didn't move a muscle when, in the morning, the "Turk," the most feared person in any training camp for players on the bubble, came up to give Baker the bad news about his release with the directive to report to Parcells with his playbook. Bavaro was out cold. The football gods were looking out for him because no morning practice was scheduled following the night off. It was a rare sign of compassion from Parcells. But Bavaro slept right through the morning team meeting before lunch.

"We had a big practice in the afternoon," he said. "I limped my way over."

The locker room was so cramped and hot, Simms said, that after taking a shower following practice, he would sweat more coming out than when he went in. Bavaro dragged himself into the sweltering locker room to get dressed for practice on what was the hottest day of the summer. His teammates knew he missed the morning meeting and was hung over. They were counting the plays until he begged out of practice or collapsed, whichever came first. "They were waiting for me to throw in the towel," he said.

He ran his first few routes and was holding his own. Parcells surprisingly didn't reprimand him for missing bed check and the morning meeting or for not running crisp routes. *Okay,* he thought, *maybe I can get through this.* At the first water break, he started to get nervous and nauseous. "I looked down and I had not one drop of sweat on me," he said. *That's weird,* he thought. "I knew that was not good."

He was completely dehydrated, and the heat was unbearable. He drank what seemed like a gallon of water trying to get fluid in his system. "I drank so much water it was sloshing around in my stomach like it wasn't going through the rest of my body," he said. "Something's wrong. And once I got it in my head that something was wrong, I knew I probably couldn't and shouldn't do it."

He was a rookie one week into training camp with the veterans, however, and tried to power through. He didn't have a roster spot guaranteed and needed to stay on the field to make the team. He ran a few more routes, but even a tough guy like Bavaro would succumb to trying to play football in stifling heat twelve hours after drinking way too much alcohol. "Ronnie, Ronnie," he yelled over to Barnes. "I think I got heat exhaustion or something."

Barnes took Bavaro's arm and placed it over his shoulder to escort him into the locker room, which was right next to the practice field. First they had to walk by Parcells, who misses nothing. Barnes was beloved by the players, and he was sympathetic to the stress their bodies endured, so he always had their backs. But he could not protect Bavaro from the coach this time.

"Heat exhaustion, coach," Barnes said as they got within a couple feet of Parcells.

"It's not heat exhaustion," Parcells barked. "He's *fucking drunk.*"

Bavaro's next two steps took him closer to the locker room but also closer to where Parcells was standing. Then an uncontrollable wave of nausea came over him, a tsunami rising up from his stomach and out his mouth.

"All the water came out," Bavaro recalled.

"He threw up," Parcells remembered.

"It splashed on Bill's shoes," Bavaro said. "*Oh, God.*"

"It might have," Parcells said with a smirk.

They were in agreement: Bavaro threw up on Parcells.

Of all the individual achievements in what is now more than a hundred years of the NFL, this was a first: a player, a rookie no less, battling a really bad hangover, barfing on a future Hall of Fame coach who controlled his football career. This was Flounder throwing up on Dean Wormer in *Animal House*. The difference is Flounder was tossed from Faber College, whereas Parcells tossed some kindness Bavaro's way and let the rookie off the hook. They later won two Super Bowls together and were inducted into the Ring of Honor one year apart.

Before he became a softie in his early eighties, Parcells was a toughie. So it was surprising that he didn't discipline or fine Bavaro, or even require him to buy a new pair of cleats. He let him slide even though it would be weeks before Parcells knew the Giants had found a gem in the fourth round. Perhaps as a make-up call later in Bavaro's career, Parcells fined him $500 for getting on the team bus to the airport with no socks, a violation of the road trip dress code. Bavaro had the required jacket and tie, but that wasn't good enough.

After he threw up on Parcells, Bavaro was escorted by Barnes to the locker room, and the trainers attempted to load him up with IV fluids but had trouble finding a vein and gave up. The only thing about Bavaro that ticked off Parcells during his first training camp was that he was giving highly respected tight ends coach Mike Pope a hard time over the instruction he was receiving.

"He was not treating Mike the right way," Parcells said. "And I talked to him about that. I said, 'Look, all this fucking guy is trying to do is help you. And here you are being an asshole. That's not right.' So, he straightened up right away."

Bavaro went to the team meeting the evening he barfed on his head coach and was still looking and feeling bad. Pope helped get him back on track.

"Don't worry," Pope said. "Sometimes things like this will endear you to your teammates."

"Really?" Bavaro said.

Bavaro did what the rest of the team only dreamed about doing during one of Parcells's typically difficult summer practices. Parcells, especially in his overweight days when the former college linebacker would act like a dictator with a whistle in his mouth, his stomach hanging over the beltline of his coach's shorts, pushed his players to their limits, keeping them banging helmets against their friends twice a day in practice.

Bavaro found it hard to believe that two months past his twenty-second birthday, he had just embarrassed himself in front of his head coach, and now his position coach was telling him that maybe it was a good thing. Pope was a nice man who later would coach personalities as diverse as ultimate wild child Jeremy Shockey and Jason Witten, winner of the Walter Payton NFL Man of the Year Award. Bavaro learned his lesson. He cut back on his drinking, and when he would drink, it was only at home. The lifestyle change may have saved his career.

"I had sowed my oats in college, and I got to the Giants and I knew I was in a situation that I was in over my head," he said. "I was just hanging on for my dear life. Going out and carousing, I knew it was going to hurt me, especially from my experience in camp."

Parcells called Bavaro the Giants' most impressive rookie of the summer. When Mowatt suffered a season-ending knee injury prior to the opener in Philadelphia, Bavaro was elevated to first team. He caught one pass in his NFL debut, a 26-yard touchdown from Simms in New York's 16–10 victory. Later in the season, Simms threw for a team-record 513 yards, and Bavaro caught twelve passes for 176 yards in a 35–30 loss to the Bengals. Bavaro finished his rookie season with thirty-seven catches for 511 yards and four touchdowns as New York made it to the second round of the playoffs.

====

"UP UNTIL I was about forty-five, I was good," Bavaro said. "I had problems, but they didn't get in the way of things. I was able to run and lift and work out. You know, I was pretty good. But after forty-five, things really started to go downhill."

The Bavaro family didn't have a history of heart problems, and Mark took the news hard that his was malfunctioning and needed an ablation procedure in 2015. "Shit," he thought. "I'm getting old." Add in neck and back problems, and he had sacrificed his body for the game he loved to play. "There is something about being treated like shit that gave you grit," he said.

Bavaro's road to recovery from Covid included many twists. A chance conversation with a longtime Giants employee helped guide him to the NFL Trust program at Massachusetts General Hospital at the end of September 2021. He was prescribed new meds that helped calm his "out-of-whack" nervous system and new psychiatrists with whom he found a connection. Six weeks later, he began to feel better.

"I think that saved my life because I was teetering on the edge," he said.

During his most helpless moments, doctors had been telling him to relax and try breathing exercises. "I said, 'Breathing exercises? My fucking body is on fire. Breathing exercises aren't going to help.'"

Lexapro, Zoloft, Celexa. Bavaro can recite just about every anti-depressant and the one thing they had in common: "None of them worked," he said. "They made things worse." His body would tremble and almost convulse from anxiety. He was given anti-seizure medication. He was given Lyrica for his nerves, propranolol to control his accelerated heart rate. The new doctors gave him lamotrigine to treat seizures. He believes the fall in the bathroom caused his neck to pinch his brain stem. He couldn't move his neck or sleep. Trazodone helped.

Before the new meds had time to kick in, his anxiety was raging through his body and mind. Susan insisted on an October trip to the ER. It was a Friday at one o'clock when he and Susan left for Boston, and the traffic was a mess. Bavaro knew the longer he waited, the longer it would take to get downtown, so he finally gave in but was freaking out right away. "I couldn't sit in a car," he said. "It's going to be a nightmare. I'm going to be sitting in traffic for God knows how long. An hour. I'll lose my mind. I can't do it."

He was having a panic attack. "Whatever caused anxiety in my brain was just going off for some reason," he said. "It affected my emotions so bad. I've never felt that alone, that hopeless. I mean, it even affected my faith. I didn't feel any presence of God. I felt total abandonment. No hope." He was crying. He cried all the time. "I was afraid of everything. Everything was a worst-case scenario," he said. "I was afraid to go in the car."

Bavaro relayed his irrational fears to Susan: *What happens if the car breaks down on the way to the hospital and we are stuck in 90-degree heat on the side of the road?* He convinced himself his body couldn't handle it. "My brain will boil," he told her. It was a very hot July and August in New England, and he tied himself in knots worrying the air conditioner in his house was about to shut down. "I'm going to fry," he told her. "I'm going to boil alive."

He ran to his computer and Googled cooler places within driving distance. He found a town one hour north where it was 75 degrees instead of 95. They would pass New Hampshire and Vermont off to the west and find a hotel in Maine. He had it all figured out. The AC, of course, operated just fine all summer. And his car did not break down on the ride to Mass General.

He was admitted to the emergency room at 2:30 p.m.

"Sedate me, do something," he pleaded with doctors.

It wasn't until 10 p.m. that he was given Ativan to calm his anxiety and agitation, but fortunately the medication he had taken at home had finally kicked in right around the time he arrived at the ER. An MRI at the hospital showed micro-hemorrhaging in his brain, which irritated the scar tissue doctors told him may have been caused by football injuries and exacerbated by the fall in the bathroom, triggering the dizziness caused by Covid. "I told the doctor I had not had to take Seroquel, and I would get so proud," he said. "The psychiatrist said, 'You're supposed to take it, Mark. You're not supposed to be running into brick walls, and it's not an accomplishment that you don't need it but you suffer through it.' I had been so conditioned to tough it out. He told me the medicine was there to help."

About the only semi-humorous moment in the ER came when he received the results of the blood tests taken by the nurses. Marijuana is legal in Massachusetts, and there are huge advertisements for cannabis dispensaries on highway billboards. Susan purchased marijuana tincture to be consumed in a dropper to relax him, and it was still in his system.

"The blood test said cannabis positive," Bavaro said.

He smoked weed at Notre Dame and gave it up. He didn't like it. The positive test at the hospital made him laugh.

By the end of 2021, Bavaro had tapered off all his medications but lamotrigine. "It's anti-seizure, antianxiety, and it's a drug they give you for manic depression," he said. "But it lets you keep the happiness part."

When Bavaro arrived in the emergency room that afternoon in October, there was a notation on his medical chart that instantly grabbed the attention of every nurse and every doctor who would treat him. "It was under the flag of self-harm," he said.

There had been dark thoughts going through Bavaro's mind he couldn't stop. "It was almost like I was hearing outside voices," he said. "It was an insidious virus and it was attacking me."

Bavaro's curiosity about suicide prior to Covid was out of sympathy for his friends and trying to understand why. Now these thoughts were real to him, and just like when half the 49ers defense, including future Hall of Famer Ronnie Lott, tried to bring him down in San Francisco in the most memorable play of the 1986 season, he refused to go down.

Super Bowl Sunday, Pasadena, California, January 25, 1987

Bavaro's second season with the Giants was the championship run. He was a first-team All-Pro, and in the Super Bowl, he didn't disappoint. He scored the go-ahead touchdown when he caught a 13-yard pass from Simms on the first possession of the third quarter. After Raul Allegre hit a 21-yard field goal the next time the Giants had the ball, the Giants took control on their third possession of the third quarter. Phil McConkey, catching a deep pass on a trick play, saw nothing but the Rose Bowl's luscious green grass and the end zone in front of him. The play went for 44 yards, but McConkey was stopped 1 yard short of the end zone when Giants former first-round pick Mark Haynes brought him down. McConkey was in agony he didn't score and lay spread-eagle on the field. Morris scored on the next play as the Giants began to run away at 26–10.

"When I was a little boy, I wanted to score a touchdown in the Super Bowl and be a pilot," said McConkey, the Naval Academy graduate. "That's all I wanted."

He thought he had blown his chance until Bavaro gifted him an easy one. Simms fired a fastball from the 6-yard line early in the fourth quarter that went right through Bavaro's hands in the end zone, hit him in the facemask and floated to McConkey, who then jumped in Bavaro's arms with the much bigger tight end lifting him up.

Bavaro had already scored, the Giants were up 33–10, and his closest friend on the team and road roommate prevented him from getting yelled at by Parcells. All was good. "I was happy for him, and he was happy because it was his dream to score a touchdown in the Super Bowl," Bavaro said.

Then he laughed.

"I would have rather caught it myself and scored two touchdowns," he said.

McConkey perfected landing navy helicopters, with their rotor blades spinning, onto the deck of small ships with only twelve feet to spare. "It was scary," he said.

It was also thrilling. Catching the touchdown in the Super Bowl after it bounced off Bavaro was the other bucket list item he was able to check off. It was no less exhilarating. As the ball floated down, McConkey said his mind raced back to when he was six years old in Buffalo tracking snowflakes into his mouth. "That's what it felt like," McConkey said.

He celebrated then with his friends. He celebrated even more with his football friends in the end zone. "Total delirium," he said.

McConkey owed that touchdown to Bavaro. But in the later years of Bavaro's life, McConkey found a way to return the favor.

Mark Bavaro's living room, Boxford, Massachusetts, February 2022

Word of Bavaro's health issues spread among the '86 Giants. He heard from Carson, the captain. Parcells called to check up on him. And McConkey, his best friend on the team, called all the time. He and McConkey talked about the future.

After a business trip to New York in the spring of 2022, McConkey met up with his wife, who was running in the Boston Marathon, and they drove to Massachusetts to visit with Bavaro and his wife in Boxford. "The son of a bitch never complains," McConkey said of Bavaro. "He never bitches. He's always grateful. He's an incredible human being and unlike anyone I've ever met in my life."

Bavaro never felt the need to go into detail with McConkey about the nights he sat in his living room and wondered whether he would have been better off dead. McConkey could have related. He had been diagnosed with tinnitus, an unbearable ringing in his ears likely caused by the combination of flying helicopters in the navy and concussions he suffered playing football in the NFL. His mind even wandered to the kid who threw a rock from across the street that hit him in the head as he was walking to his first day of kindergarten. It sent him to the hospital, and decades later McConkey wondered whether that contributed to the ringing in his ears. The tinnitus he'd developed in 2020 was ruining his life. It was only after months of suffering that he was able to find some relief.

"I remember one night I woke up and I was like, holy shit, it's like somebody sounded an alarm in my ears," McConkey said. "It was so loud it kept me up at night. It came on so hard and it was so constant. I saw my doctor, who said there was no cure."

It was excruciating. McConkey couldn't imagine going through the rest of his life with his ears ringing 24/7. "It was the only time, the first time in my life, where I thought, if my life ended, I'd be okay," he said. "It was horrible. It's not that I contemplated at all doing anything to expedite it."

If the ringing was eight on a scale of one to ten, it's down to a three. McConkey found an audiologist through a local newspaper in La Jolla who treats tinnitus and then a doctor who he is not even sure is a doctor who also suffered from tinnitus. Between the audiologist and doctor, McConkey is on a regimen of vitamins, is meditating for the first time in his life, and wears hearing aids. Outside noise also helps drown out the ringing. The problem has been reduced to where he can live with it. "It's horrific and people commit suicide routinely from this," he said. "Before this, never did I think it would be a good thing for my life to end."

McConkey has been aggressive parlaying his Naval Academy education and his NFL playing career into a second career in the financial world and is one of the '86 Giants success stories. McConkey was offered a job on Parcells's coaching staff in 1990 after his final year in the NFL but turned it down. He briefly tried politics in New Jersey but lost a Republican primary for a seat in Congress. He focused for more than thirty years on business and has involved Bavaro in some of his ventures, including his current job at Academy Securities, based in San Diego, where McConkey is president. Bavaro has struggled to find a satisfying career in his life following football after also deciding not to pursue a coaching career. He's involved in a business venture with former teammates Lawrence Taylor and Ottis Anderson, but he has never settled into a long-term career after football.

McConkey is frustrated by former teammates who have not found a way to transfer the same passion that made them great football players into their life after football.

"It's not just Mark's issue. The majority of guys, at least that I played with, feel the same way. I don't understand it," he said. "I've had three careers in my life, the military, professional sports, and business. These are some of the most competitive people on the face of the planet. Just take that and put it over here. But they're unfamiliar with business or starting a business or being an entrepreneur. They shy away from it and do what they're comfortable with. They don't try, or they're somewhat intimidated. And it's like, you're the most fearless person I've ever known. How many times did you get up after getting your ass kicked on the football field? Time and time again, that's why you made it in the NFL. Why don't they take that incredible competitive spirit and direct it toward business?"

McConkey doesn't blame this solely on the players. Football is all they've known. They were told they were the best in high school when they received college scholarships. They were told that again in college when they were about to be drafted. They've been told that in the NFL. They were trained to be football players, not CEOs. They thrived in a protected football environment with abnormally high-paying first jobs. Once they are used up by the NFL, either by diminishing skills or injury, they are often lost. McConkey doesn't believe players get enough assistance from their teams in adapting to their new life.

"That's something that the NFL sucks at and the Players Association sucks at," he said. "They don't do anything. Once you're done, nobody gives a shit. Even Mark Bavaro, as popular and legendary as that guy is, nobody gives a fucking shit." Gary Reasons, a starter at linebacker on the Giants' first two Super Bowl teams, benefited from the exposure of playing with Taylor, Banks, and Carson. He played eight years with the Giants, finished up with one year with the Bengals in 1992, and had the ambition to parlay his experiences into the post-football career McConkey hoped would happen for all his teammates.

"Once you are accustomed to having that trophy be a part of your life, it can really set you in motion for planning for success and transitioning into the real world," Reasons said.

Bavaro did reach out after Parcells returned to New York with the Jets in 1997 and asked whether he could give coaching a trial run in training camp. Parcells always takes care of his former players and welcomed Bavaro with open arms. He spent the summer helping to coach tight ends. He had been running a football camp for fifteen years with his younger brother David, who had a five-year career as a linebacker with four NFL teams, and it left him wanting more.

"I miss football, I'm not doing anything, I'm not good at anything, I never learned to do anything," he said. "I was making money. But I was thinking, 'I need a career, I need something.'"

One camp was enough to convince Bavaro coaching was not for him. He hated it. The hours were long, there was too much film to watch, he didn't like the insensitivity that went into cutting players, and he was shocked by the "infighting in the coaches' meetings," although most of the Jets crew had previously worked for Parcells with the Giants and Patriots. At the end of the summer of '97, he sat down with Parcells to evaluate the experience.

"What do you think?" Parcells said.

"I don't think this is for me," Bavaro said.

Parcells smiled.

"Good," he said.

Parcells knew if Bavaro wasn't all-in, coaching would be a miserable life. Bavaro learned that summer that Parcells is even tougher on his assistants than he is on his players. "I don't think he wanted to have me as somebody he was going to have to shit on," Bavaro said. "He didn't want our relationship to turn into that. He was happy when I said no."

Bavaro thanked Parcells for the opportunity, got up from his chair, left his office, and never looked back. He has no way of knowing how his relationship with Parcells might have changed if he worked on his staff . . . only that it would have changed.

He's thankful he has a great friendship with Parcells, knows he can lean on him for advice and support, and that long ago he forgave him for throwing up on his shoes.

Parcells has forgiven other players for a lot worse.

3

L.T. AND LAWRENCE

L awrence Taylor and Joe Namath are New York football royalty. But their legacies are tarnished.

Namath's addiction to alcohol played out in public during an ESPN broadcast in 2003 when he was interviewed on the New York Jets sideline by Suzy Kolber and pathetically told her on camera he wanted to kiss her right then and there. Kolber brushed aside his uncomfortable advance, and Namath later admitted he was drunk. He says he's not had alcohol since that humiliating incident and credits it with saving his life, because he was on the way to drinking himself to death.

"I still have a fear for what that stuff does to me and what it could do to me," Namath said in an interview with Graham Bensinger.

Taylor was in and out of drug rehabilitation centers for his addiction to cocaine during and after his thirteen-year career with the Giants. A second positive drug test that resulted in a four-game suspension to begin the 1988 season was when he hit rock bottom during his playing days, but he's suffered through equally low moments in his life after football. He managed not to test positive the last five years of his career, when he supposedly stayed clean, knowing a third positive could have gotten him kicked out of the NFL. But he was back on crack right after his retirement following the 1993 season. Multiple drug-related arrests among other indiscretions after he retired kept his name in the news for way too many cringeworthy incidents.

Joe Namath. Broadway Joe.

Lawrence Taylor. L.T.

Namath and Taylor are fighting off the demons built by their stage names. Addicts are never cured. They are always in recovery and take their sobriety one day at a time. Namath and Taylor have that in common, in addition to being the most iconic players in New York football history. Namath was the MVP of Super Bowl III, following through on his guarantee that the upstart Jets from the AFL would defeat the powerful Baltimore Colts of the mighty NFL. Taylor is simply the best defensive player in NFL history and led the Giants to two Super Bowl victories.

Taylor could be loud and obnoxious in the locker room, but it was all in good fun, and he was popular with his teammates, even if he scared the crap out of many of them. It was after he left the locker room that he got himself in trouble doing business with degenerate drug dealers who were happy to accommodate his needs and take his money. "I know Lawrence Taylor the man," Harry Carson said. "I know he's a sweetheart of a guy if you get to know him. I still say I'm glad I'm not him."

Taylor, who now lives in South Florida, is among the major attractions at Namath's annual charity golf tournament at the scenic Old Palm Golf Club in Palm Beach Gardens. After getting in eighteen holes in March 2022, Taylor skipped lunch and the accompanying auction of sports memorabilia for the rich folk who paid to play with the celebrities. Instead, he is relaxing on the veranda overlooking the course. He appears happy and healthy, which hasn't always been the case. His completely gray beard makes him look a little older than his sixty-three years, having celebrated his birthday one month earlier. He attempted to remedy that after he saw former Cowboys defensive end Ed "Too Tall" Jones at a golf tournament a few weeks earlier and asked him about his black beard, which was gray the last time they saw each other on the former NFL players charity golf circuit. Jones let him in on his secret, and Taylor bought the hair color kit Jones recommended and applied it. "My face broke out in a rash," he said, laughing. "Damn Too Tall."

Taylor has an old friend by his side who drives him around, and he has a new lady interest he is crazy about. His first two marriages ended in divorce, and his third divorce was imminent. Having a driver was a smart idea for Taylor and others on the road. He was arrested for DUI on a Florida highway in 2016 and pled guilty in 2017. He was stopped after he allegedly crashed into a motorhome and sideswiped a trooper's patrol car. After he was wobbly on a field sobriety test, he was handcuffed. "Why, why?" he pleaded with the officers. Five hours later, tests showed blood alcohol levels of 0.082 and 0.084, barely above the Florida limit of 0.08. He was given one year of probation, and his driver's license was suspended for nine months.

Those days, he hopes, are behind him.

L.T. lights up a big cigar that envelops him in smoke but insists it's the only thing he smokes in his early sixties. Taylor said he has been drug-free since 1998, the last time he was in a drug rehabilitation center, which came after arrests that fall for buying crack in Florida and possessing drugs in New Jersey.

"I've been clean ever since," Taylor said.

He knows those are literally the famous last words of addicts.

"I don't even really think about it," he said. "It just doesn't come up in my conversations. I am not going to get caught up in that life again."

That's quite a difference in how he summed up life from the cocaine-snorting and crack-smoking days. "I saw coke as the only bright spot in my future," he said on CBS's *60 Minutes* in 2004. "I had gotten really bad. I mean, my place was almost like a crack house, not where you sold it, but I had a lot of stuff in my house." The only people he wanted to interact with, he told *60 Minutes*, were addicts, dealers, and prostitutes. At one time, he was spending $1,000 a day on his habits.

Taylor was elected to the Pro Football Hall of Fame in his first year of eligibility in 1999. Hall of Fame bylaws mandate that off-the-field conduct is not to be considered when judging a candidate's worthiness, but many of the old-school selectors refused to vote for him anyway. He still received the support required to make it to the final four modern-era candidates and then the 80 percent minimum vote to receive his gold jacket.

Taylor has by no means stayed trouble-free since his induction, even if he is to be taken at his word that he has not used drugs this century. In particular, there was a disturbing case in 2010 of Taylor being arrested for rape and prostitution charges in a case involving an underage girl at a cheap hotel in Rockland County outside New York City. He insisted the girl told him she was nineteen. The Associated Press reported ten months later that Taylor "pleaded guilty to sexual misconduct and having sex with a sixteen-year-old he thought was a prostitute." The girl denied she was a prostitute and said she was forced to go to Taylor's hotel room in Montebello, New York. He was required to register as a sex offender.

He was arrested in 2021 in Florida when he moved out of the house he shared with his third wife, Lynette, presumably to avoid any confrontations—he says local law enforcement encouraged the move. But he failed to inform the proper authorities he was relocating down the street to a hotel, a violation of the laws applied to registered sex offenders. It was cleared up months later without any significant penalty. Immediately after the judge said he was free to leave, Taylor went from the courthouse to the golf course, which has always been his sanctuary.

Life after football has been much better for Taylor in his sixties than at any other time since he retired. "A lot of us go through problems," he said. "You're on top and then all of a sudden it stops. Where do you go from there? That's the hardest part. It's tough." As long as he continues to keep his name out of the newspaper for the wrong reasons, he can generate income by making appearances at memorabilia shows. "I'm still in demand. I can be comfortable," he said. The money was so much different when he played. Taylor held out all of training camp in 1990 until the Wednesday before the opening game of the season before agreeing to a three-year, $4.5 million contract. Of course, on just a couple days of practice, he played in the Sunday night opener against the Eagles and sacked Randall Cunningham three times. In his final season in 1993, he made a career-high $2.8 million. If he was a free agent today, coming off production similar to his 1986 MVP and Super Bowl season when he led the NFL with 20.5 sacks, his contract would be worth more than the $150 million the Giants were valued at in the early '90s. How much would he get in today's market? "It would be Giants *and* Taylor Stadium," he said. Instead, his base salary post–Super Bowl in 1987 was $900,000 rather than the $40 million annual pay he would command today.

When I visited Taylor at his home in Upper Saddle River, New Jersey, in December 1998, his life was out of control. He sat in a cloud of cigar smoke—some things never change—and we discussed the turbulence of his first five years of retirement. He had recently returned home after a forty-eight-day stay in Honesty House, a drug rehabilitation facility in Sterling, New Jersey. It was the beginning of his sobriety, which he says continues to this day.

He will never be a Boy Scout and knows he's one weak moment from getting back into the life he no longer wants. "I'm an addict regardless," he said that day at his house. "If I've been clean for one day or a thousand years, I'm a recovering addict, and that possibility is always going to be there. There is no guarantee about that."

Taylor did not travel in the same circles as his teammates except for wide receiver Bobby Johnson, who made a heroic, crucial fourth-down catch in 1986 in a victory in Minnesota. He shared with Taylor an affinity for crack, which prompted Parcells to trade him to San Diego during training camp the following summer. Taylor's stature dictated patience from Parcells. Johnson's did not.

Taylor and Simms were the faces of the franchise, but the only place they saw each other off the field was the golf course and players-only dinners. "I don't even know how to explain my relationship with

Lawrence," Simms said. "It's not like we ever did hang out or anything. I don't know if he liked me at first, but when we started getting our team together, I think our relationship changed for sure."

Simms was married with a one-year-old son when Taylor joined the Giants. They didn't have much in common other than being incredibly competitive. "You know, I think the greatest decision I ever made about Lawrence was one day, we're in the locker room and he looked at me and he goes, 'Do you want to go out with us?' And I said, 'Oh, you know,' and I really waited. I said, 'No, I don't think I will.' And he just looks at me and goes, 'Good decision.' And he walks out."

Former teammates are skeptical of Taylor's claims of abstinence but still hopeful that they might be true. "I'm quite sure, as long as I'm alive, there is always going to be some controversy with me," Taylor said in 1998. "People must think I get up in the morning and say, 'Let me see, what can I get into now?'"

He wakes up in the morning today with his golf clubs nearby, choosing whether to play eighteen, thirty-six, or fifty-four holes. His loud cackle at Namath's tournament is reminiscent of a simpler time in his life back in his rookie year in 1981 when he was a confident and respectful twenty-two-year-old with an infectious personality. He immediately impressed the coaches by covering 1.75 miles in the twelve-minute conditioning run to open camp and then belting out "She'll Be Coming 'Round the Mountain," in the dining hall to fulfill the rookie ritual.

"I don't know the words to many songs," he said.

The next day he looked over the grounds of Pace University, saw a couple of horses grazing, and decided his song really should have been "Old MacDonald."

That summer, following home preseason games at Giants Stadium, Taylor often showed up at the Front Row, a bar on Paterson Plank Road owned by former Giants guard Doug Van Horn, less than five minutes from the stadium. It was the unofficial hangout for players and the younger beat writers covering the team. What was seen and heard on those Saturday nights was off the record but stored away for future use. Taylor would arrive early, stay late, and always had a drink in his hand. He was outgoing and had quickly established himself as the best player on the team, and that quickly turned him into the bar's number-one attraction.

He loved it.

That was innocent enough.

The trouble began when he was first introduced to cocaine at a party during his rookie season. Two years later, he was doing crack. Although he promises he never played a game high and teammates say they never saw him doing drugs around the team, Taylor did admit to going on binges the night before games and was fuzzy on details as to whether he got high hours before kickoff before he arrived at the stadium. "I'm not going to say I never had, but I just don't remember," he said. "I wouldn't remember that."

He pushed back against any suggestion that he hid in the corner of the locker room or inside a stall in the bathroom to snort coke with a rolled-up dollar bill thirty minutes before a game. "No, no, no. I would never bring drugs into the locker room," he said. "That wouldn't happen. If I'm willing to do drugs, it's going to be after the game or maybe the night before."

How often did that happen?

Taylor smiled. "I may have hung out a couple of times," he said.

The stats make the question seem ludicrous. If he wasn't a drug addict, could he have been even better, even more unstoppable, won more Super Bowls?

Stats and honors: Pro Football Hall of Fame, two-time Super Bowl champion, 142 career sacks, NFL MVP, three-time Defensive Player of the Year, Defensive Rookie of the Year, eight-time first-team All-Pro, ten Pro Bowls, named to NFL's Seventy-Fifth and One Hundredth Anniversary All-Time Team, Giants Ring of Honor, No. 56 retired.

One award he could never win: NFL Man of the Year. It has annually recognized a player for excellence on and off the field since 1970 and was renamed in 1999 for the late Walter Payton, a Taylor contemporary. "My legacy is going to be messed up," Taylor said. "But I still think I'm one of the best players that played the game."

He dominated from the first day of training camp in 1981. Then–head coach Ray Perkins and defensive coordinator Bill Parcells declared they were going to make Taylor fight for a starting job even though he was the second overall pick of the draft on a dreadful team. It took one play, maybe two, for Perkins and Parcells to look at each other and realize they had to elevate him to the first-team defense ahead of journeyman John Skorupan at right outside linebacker or they would lose all credibility with the team.

Could Taylor have dominated even more if he had taken better care of himself? He was already terrorizing quarterbacks. He had such incredible strength he snapped Joe Theismann's lower leg in half in a 1985 *Monday Night Football* game, ending the Washington quarterback's career. Theismann clearly doesn't hold a grudge. Taylor autographed a jersey for him, and it hangs in Theismann's living room. The loud snap and grotesque bending of Theismann's leg made L.T. lose his composure: he waved frantically for the doctors to rush onto the field and then he held his head in his hands. Footage of this moment has become so famous that it appeared in the Oscar-nominated movie *The Blind Side.*

Taylor was as fearsome as any defender in league history. Still, one teammate said that although Taylor was named first-team All-Pro in 1984 and 1985, and he made big plays with double-digit sacks each year, his lifestyle negatively impacted his week-to-week dominance. The teammate believes he earned his postseason honors those two seasons on reputation, but he bounced back in 1986 to win the league MVP award.

Taylor thought about how his thirteen-year career might have played out if he had indeed lived a clean life like Simms. "I could have been better. I could have been worse," he said. "They were saying in life you may not be able to handle things, but on the football field you control things. That's my domain, that's where I live. Could I have been a better player? I could have, but who knows? I am what I am."

Considering the short careers of drug addicts in the NFL, Taylor managed to play thirteen years without imploding. That is not to be celebrated, but it does say something about how much he loved to play. It's also hard to find a teammate who resents him. "Lawrence is a member of the family," George Martin said. "He's not the only one with warts. We all have imperfections."

Burt came to the Giants in 1981, the same year as Taylor, and he was never afraid to open his mouth to him. They had that kind of relationship despite Burt being a replaceable part, an undrafted free agent, and Taylor being irreplaceable. Burt knows where Taylor could have taken his game without drugs. "He achieved a lot when he was in the NFL. He could have achieved so much more," he said. "The first time I saw him, I'm like, what a freaking physical specimen."

Taylor may have stayed clean on game day, but Burt does not discount the damage he did the rest of the week. "What about the other six days that affected his body and his play?" he said. "He was great. Listen, he was a dog. On Sunday, he played his ass off. You have to understand Lawrence. When you do drugs and alcohol for that period of time, it changes your body chemistry. He is a really good guy, but when he came here they had the old crew of players, and he gravitated toward those guys. He was a magnet toward those guys. They gave him a lot of bad habits. He was a drinker before when he was in college. But as time went on, his brain just started warping from the alcohol and drugs. When I see him, he knows that I know. There's nowhere to go and hide from me."

If the Taylor who turned sixty in 2019 could have a talk with twenty-four-year-old Lawrence Taylor, he knows exactly what he would say. "I think everybody should stay away from drugs," he said.

He may not want to be the hard-partying L.T. now, but he embraced that lifestyle when he played, and it doesn't sound like he would want that to change if given the option to do it all again. "Drugs and drinking and the women, those are the type of things that made me who I am today," he said. "I'm not a choirboy. I think about it. If I would have stayed in the gym and had a better reputation, I might have been a better person. But who would know me? Nobody would even know me. Who the fuck would know me? Who's that guy who played for the Giants? He's a good athlete, but he's just boring."

I read Taylor something he said to me in 2017:

My health is not the best. I am surprised at the things I cannot do now. I can't walk for long or everything aches. That's basically all I can say about it. Your mind is not the same. Sometimes I wake up and can't remember what I did the day before. It comes in spurts. Sometimes I can remember everything. Sometimes I can't remember shit. You know whatever you want to do has limitations.

Here was his reaction to that quote in March 2022:

That's pretty much it. I do forget a lot. I don't handle anything right now that's important. This is a function of age, and hell, I look at it and I've taken a lot of hits in the NFL. I don't consider myself a dormant person, but it's taken its toll. My joints hurt. My ankles hurt. I get gout now. I can't concentrate on anything for too much time. I'm going to one thing then going to another thing. But as far as health-wise, other than I probably need to lose a couple of pounds, I'm good.

Taylor played at 245 pounds. He's up to 261.

He doesn't spend his time worrying about how many concussions he had in the NFL and what impact it's had on his brain. He's not reading up on CTE. "I don't know enough about it," he said. "I don't consider myself a scholar, and if I wasn't a scholar before it happened, I ain't going to be a scholar now because I ain't going to take the time to read about it. The good thing is I'm surrounded by a lot of good people and they make sure I stay on point."

Taylor is content now being Lawrence Taylor, golf addict. In the 2004 interview with *60 Minutes*, he said, "L.T. left a long time ago. He's left the building. . . . I don't want to be L.T. no more. L.T. is good for the comic books. I like Lawrence Taylor. Lawrence Taylor can handle life a lot better than L.T. L.T. can play some helluva football, though, he's a helluva football player."

Carson implored Taylor through the years to do away with L.T., the trouble-seeking alter ego. "L.T. is a bad-ass. Get rid of L.T.," Carson still says now. "You need to let L.T. commit suicide and just be Lawrence Taylor. L.T. is what got him into trouble. Most people know him or recognize him as L.T. So how do you stop being L.T. to people who want to continue to call you that? L.T. was a drag on his life. I know the real Lawrence Taylor, and I just want him to take good care of himself."

It took forever, but Taylor insists he's ditched his evil twin. "L.T. left the building a long time ago. There wasn't enough excitement in my life for him. He said, 'Fuck you, I'm out of here,'" Taylor said. "Now I'm just Lawrence."

When I listed his 1986 teammates so distraught over health or drug issues that they considered suicide in the years since Super Bowl XXI, Taylor was unaware and taken aback. He volunteered despite all his troubles that he never once thought about taking his own life. Unlike some teammates who believe brain trauma from their football career led to depression and suicidal thoughts, all of Taylor's problems have been self-inflicted and not related to football injuries. "I've gone through a lot of shit," he said. "I'm confident in myself that I can pull my way out of it. Right now, there hasn't been an instance where I wanted to take my own life because of some bullshit. Everybody is trying to get that CTE checked, of course. But I can't say that I've ever wanted to just go out and kill myself. I've been down before. I've made bad decisions. A lot of them. But I'd rather be living." Carson was critical of Taylor's lifestyle in the years after L.T.'s career ended when he was more interested in cocaine than making something of his life after football. "It got back to him and he was angry," Carson said.

They had a good relationship in the eight years they played together, but Carson's comments led to a lengthy period where Taylor shut him out of his life. He refused to invite him to attend his Hall of Fame induction.

"Did you get an invitation?" George Martin asked Carson.

"No, but I'm going," Carson said.

Carson arrived in Canton with his wife Maribel and was sitting among the sun-drenched crowd in folding chairs at the bottom of the steps in front of the Hall of Fame. Taylor was with the other Hall of Famers on the podium and didn't realize at first that Carson was there. During one of the ESPN commercial breaks before Taylor's speech, host Chris Berman introduced Carson and he stood up and waved. On the stage, Taylor heard the introduction, got to his feet, saw Carson and smiled. All was forgiven.

"You know, me and this guy, we had some words a while back and we kind of split ways and we just didn't really talk," Taylor improvised in his speech. "But I tell you, Harry Carson came out for me today, and that's the classiest thing I've ever seen in my life, Harry. Thank you, thank you. Love you, man. I love you."

When the ceremony was over, the new inductees walked off the stage and into the Hall of Fame building to mingle with each other and families and friends. "We're in the basement of the Hall of Fame and our paths cross," Carson said.

It was an awkward moment, the two of them making eye contact, and the ice needed to be broken.

As Carson tells this story in his home in Upper Saddle River, Maribel enters the room.

"What happens, Maribel?" Carson said to her.

"Lawrence hugs Harry and is just sobbing on his shoulder," she said.

"Like four minutes," Carson said.

"It was an uncomfortable moment for the rest of us who are watching because it felt so personal. And unexpected," Maribel said. "I sort of wanted to disappear and give them that moment."

"Nobody would disturb us," Carson said.

"It was a moment," Maribel said.

"I certainly wasn't expecting it, but I welcomed it," Carson said.

It was a soft side of Lawrence Taylor few have ever seen.

═══

WHEN TAYLOR ARRIVED in New York in 1981, Parcells was the defensive coordinator, and Belichick was the linebackers and special teams coach. He had incredible talent and two of the great defensive coaches of all time teaching him the nuances of the professional game.

"I loved coaching L.T.," Belichick said. "He was elite in terms of physical talent, football instincts, toughness, competitiveness. He put the team first with his unselfish play on the field. I was fortunate to have the opportunity to coach the player that every other defensive player will be compared to in the history of the game. He was simply unblockable. Anthony Muñoz was really the only player who could battle him evenly. Every offense had to figure out a way to handle him, and after a couple of years, he was able to figure out what the opponent was doing and what he needed to do about it."

Once Taylor revolutionized the game with his pass rush ability as an outside linebacker in a 3-4 defense, the inevitable comparisons began. Every year or two, the "next L.T." was predicted to be coming in the next draft, but it never happened. The position is now called edge rusher. Any way you say it, there is only one Lawrence Taylor.

After Parcells became head coach in 1983, Belichick spent more time with Taylor and devised creative ways to use him to stay ahead of offensive coordinators scheming against him. Whenever Belichick is asked about Taylor, he could go on forever, but he doesn't want to say whether he tried to assist him off the field.

"I'm not going to get into any player's personal life or my personal conversations with them," he said. "Those will remain private between us. I will say that I never had an issue with his effort on the football field. He did everything he could to help the team win and tried to play team defense. At times, his instincts overtook his assignment, and he tried to make a play that would help the team win. That worked out a high percentage of the time, but when it didn't, I would never second-guess his intentions. His defensive intelligence and awareness are second to none. He could tell me exactly what the offense was doing to him by the second series. He knew by the way the offensive players looked at him whether they were going to block him. His anticipation was tremendous."

Taylor's life in the '80s is a distant memory for him. L.T. once was asked what he remembered about his draft day in 1981. "I had forty-one Coors Lights the day I was drafted, so I couldn't tell you," he said. He was so out of control, it was impossible for his antics to surprise his friends on the team. But then he found a way to top himself. Burt and Banks have dueling handcuff stories about Taylor. Neither knew about the other story. "They could be different incidents," Banks said. "Both can be true with L.T."

Banks recalls the night before a game in Houston that Taylor came into the meeting room with a sweater covering his hands. He sat down and revealed he was handcuffed. His teammates figured he interrupted kinky sex to attend the mandatory meeting and couldn't get out of the handcuffs. There was no key and they were not gag handcuffs. Hotel security called Texas state troopers, and they pulled Taylor out of the meetings and removed the handcuffs.

"That could have happened," Burt said.

He paused. "But I know this one did."

The 9 p.m. team meeting at the Hilton Woodcliff Lake the night before a 1987 home game had broken down to offense and defense. Belichick had half a can of film to go over last-minute game planning. "Taylor walked in just in time," Burt said. "He's got a towel. He sits down and he's got the towel on his lap. I always have my eye on that guy. You don't know what the hell he's going to pull."

"What do you got over there?" Burt asked.

"Nothing," Taylor answered.

Burt pulled away the towel. Taylor was in handcuffs.

"They put handcuffs on me," Taylor said. "I got three girls in the room."

"Get the hell out of here," Burt said. "You're full of crap."

Taylor had previously sent prostitutes to wear out an opposing player the night before they were to play at Giants Stadium. Now they were returning the favor. Burt placed the towel back on Taylor's lap, and when the meeting was over Taylor got up to walk to the elevator to take him back to his room.

"I'm following you," Burt said.

They arrived at Taylor's room, and he gave Burt his key to open the door. He slid the key card in and was amazed.

"Oh my gosh," Burt said. "Three women are passed out naked. It looks like a freaking crime scene. It was unbelievable. Who knows what they're on."

Burt grabbed his shirt and wiped his fingerprints from the door. He threw the key on the floor and ran down the hallway to his room as if he was chasing Randall Cunningham. "I didn't see nothing," Burt convinced himself. "I don't know anything that is going on."

One day Simms and Taylor were walking up the tunnel in the stadium to the fenced-in grass practice field in the Giants Stadium parking lot. Simms realized Taylor was coming off a night when he was definitely L.T. Lawrence, meanwhile, was dragging as he made the long walk.

"How we doing, big boy?" Simms said.

"Oh man, Simms," Taylor moaned.

Then in the next breath, he said, "You know, there's only one thing to do today."

"Yeah, what's that?" Simms said.

"I'm just gonna go crazy," Taylor said.

And he did. "He would literally go out and wreck the practice," Simms said. "Nobody could block him. He just gets that burst of energy and did it, and, you know, that's who he was."

Burt said he knew when Taylor had been out drinking the previous evening because he came in "smelling like an old bar, a gin mill, and would be grumpy and sleepy all day. Then after practice, he would take a shower, put on a new set of clothes and be refreshed. And nobody knew where he was going."

Mark Collins remembers the night before a game in Dallas. Taylor's hotel room was right across the hall from his. Collins couldn't sleep and it was close to midnight. He walked down the hallway to buy a soda from the vending machine when the elevator doors opened. "Lawrence gets off the elevator with a twelve-pack of beer under each arm and two chicks on each side walking to his room," he said.

"What the hell?" Collins said.

"Don't tell anybody," Taylor said.

Collins presumes Taylor had a busy evening before coming out the next day at Texas Stadium and putting on a dominant performance. "I know what this man did the night before," Collins said. "Nobody could do that but this man. Nobody could do shit like that. It was unbelievable."

Several players said Wellington Mara at one point banned alcohol from being served on the team charter on the return flight from road trips. Nothing was ever served on the way out. It had gotten out of hand when the players who didn't drink passed beer and alcohol to the players who did. One player was so inebriated that his teammates put a blanket over him and paraded him off the plane with a sign, "Mr. Drunk America." After the ban was put in place, the drinkers got around it by purchasing little bottles of alcohol and either hiding them in their overnight bag or asking flight attendants to stick them in their pockets.

Parcells had rules for team meetings. No hats, no sunglasses, sit up in the chair. The desks had armchair tables. "Like the second grade," Burt said. Taylor would invariably walk into the defensive meeting room with sunglasses hiding his bloodshot eyes, curl up on the floor, and fall asleep. Taylor's wild in-season partying on Thursday nights ran into Friday mornings, which made him late for work two days before a crucial late-season game for first place in the NFC East in Washington in 1986. The winner would likely secure home field advantage throughout the playoffs and be the favorite to get to the Super Bowl.

Cranky defensive line coach Lamar Leachman called the meeting to install additional pass rush schemes. L.T. stumbled into the cramped room, crawled underneath his seat without removing his sunglasses or hat, and made himself comfortable in the fetal position. He was napping before Leachman had the lights turned off. Leachman was running the projector back and forth looking for keys to outplay Washington's dominant offensive line known as the "Hogs" and was having a hard time coming up with a creative answer. The man with the answer was fast asleep.

The lights came back on. Taylor didn't move. He had advanced to the REM stage. He was out.

"Goddamn it, Lawrence," Leachman screamed in his southern drawl. "You think you'd fucking be awake for something like this."

Taylor reluctantly opened his eyes, lifted himself off the floor, removed his sunglasses and told the coach to run the film back. He grabbed the chalk out of Leachman's hand, drew up the pass rush scheme on the blackboard and explained why it would work. Leachman and the players agreed Taylor had uncovered the key to the game. L.T. put his sunglasses back on and stared at Leachman.

"Can I fucking go back to sleep now?" he said.

And he did.

"He just saw the game differently," Banks said. "The game was slower for him. That's the difference between him and Von Miller and Khalil Mack and all the rest of them, you know? Because they can't do what he does. If they lined up and ran at Von Miller, they block Von Miller. They ran at Lawrence Taylor, you don't block Lawrence Taylor. You run at Khalil Mack, you block Khalil Mack over and over and over. Block Lawrence once, it's never happening again in that game."

Two days later, Taylor had three sacks against All-Pro left tackle Joe Jacoby, the Giants beat Washington by 10 points, took a one-game lead in the NFC East, and clinched it the next week. New York earned the NFC's No. 1 seed and overwhelmed San Francisco 49–3 and Washington 17–0 in the playoffs, and then beat Denver 39–20 in Super Bowl XXI.

"It was the most rewarding year I had in football," Taylor said. "You wonder where all the years went."

THE '86 GIANTS didn't have a legitimate opportunity to defend their championship, with a strike predicted after the second week of the 1987 season. They opened the season with a Monday night loss in Chicago in a much-hyped matchup of the previous two Super Bowl winners. The '85 Bears are considered one of the best teams of that Super Bowl era, the '86 Giants were just as good, but in 1987 the Bears beat the Giants, 34–19.

If the Giants of 1986 had played the Bears of 1985, Taylor has no doubt about the outcome. "You can talk about your '85 Bears. I don't give a shit about them," he said. "Hey, listen, we were the most dominant team. We took people apart, destroyed them."

After the opening game loss in 1987, the Giants suffered a dreadful home-opener loss to a bad Cowboys team in the second-to-last year of the Tom Landry era in Dallas. When the Giants took the field against Dallas, it was apparent it was going to be the last game they played for a while. Barring a last-minute breakthrough in labor talks between the owners and the union, the players planned to go on strike for the second time in six seasons. Unlike the 1982 strike, which lasted fifty-seven days and wiped out seven regular season games, NFL owners were not going to allow the players to shut down the industry and cost them millions of dollars in television revenue.

Even before the first picket sign was paraded in front of any of the twenty-eight team facilities, the owners canceled the games for the following weekend and implemented a strategy hatched by Cowboys president Tex Schramm to fracture the players' unity by using replacement players in week four. The quality of the games was awful—players of varying experience and ability were signed from all walks of life—but the union busting ultimately worked. Big name stars like Taylor, Joe Montana, and Danny White hurt union solidarity by eventually crossing the picket line. Result: the players called off the strike after just twenty-four days and three weeks of very bad football with the key issue of free agency still unresolved.

Giants general manager George Young held tryouts and stocked his replacement team with a bunch of truck drivers and supermarket workers with minimal football background or physical skills. Young didn't want to insult his Super Bowl champions who were walking the picket line by aggressively recruiting scabs. He put little to no effort into fielding a competitive team. Some organizations, like Washington, went all-out to bring in the best players they could find off the street, and its team was 3–0 in the replacement games with not one veteran player crossing the picket line. Just like in 1982, Washington won the Super Bowl in a strike season. The Giants were 0–3 in the strike games, even with L.T. showing up for the last one in Buffalo doubling as a linebacker and tight end. As great as L.T. was, he could not win as a one-man team. New York's 6–3 loss to the Bills set football back fifty years.

The Giants may not have brought in any replacement players they were interested in keeping, but they did bring a collection of players with questionable character.

"You had to see those tryouts," receivers coach Pat Hodgson said. "Hell, they were checking their bags for guns and stuff when they came in the stadium. There were probably drugs. When we played the first game, they were all getting their pictures taken in front of the lockers in uniform, and they stole a bunch of the equipment out of the lockers. They stole everything. None of the [regular] players had equipment when they got back. There's some funny stuff that you can't make up."

The combination of lost wages for the regular rank and file and the replacement games damaging the league's integrity put pressure on both sides to end the walkout. The free agency issue was eventually settled in court in February 1993, and it began one month later with the salary cap introduced in 1994. The ineptitude of the Giants strike team put together by Young—they lost 41–21 to the 49ers, 38–12 to Washington, before the loss in Buffalo—placed the Giants veterans in an impossible situation when the replacements handed the season back to them at 0–5. In the twenty-four days the regular players were on strike, Hodgson remembers Bill Parcells getting disgusted, losing interest, and allowing Bill Belichick to be the de facto head coach. "Big Bill was all pissed off and pouting," Hodgson said. "Little Bill did a lot of the team meetings. You saw the first changes in him being a head coach when he took over during the strike."

The replacement players were so inept that from across the field Parcells and 49ers coach Bill Walsh looked at each other and laughed. The Giants regulars came back and won six of their last ten games, but the 6–9 record left them far short of the playoffs and feeling cheated of a real chance to defend their title.

"It was a waste of a season," Collins said.

By the time the Giants reported to camp in 1988, the stench of the strike season had cleared. Any residual bad feelings from union activists on the Giants about Taylor crossing the picket line had subsided. But just as they didn't have the same team in '87 as they had in '86, they were even further removed another year later. That's life in the NFL. L.T. and Simms were their only irreplaceable players, and Taylor was about to get suspended.

Taylor had devised a system to circumvent the NFL's drug testing program, which started in 1987. When the urine collectors showed up at Giants Stadium to get him to provide his sample, he recruited teammates he was confident were clean to pee in a cup for him, and he would swap it out. One high-profile teammate admitted to me he was one of Taylor's enablers and gave him his urine several times.

"I knew he was dirty. I knew his lifestyle," the teammate said. "But I also knew he was very important to us to win."

The player would go into the stall in the Giants locker room bathroom, close the door and urinate into a cup. He left the cup on top of the back of the toilet and immediately retreated to his locker or the training room. He would let Taylor know the dirty deed with the clean pee was complete. "Lawrence would take it," he said. "I would walk away. Run away."

It was not exactly a sophisticated operation, but it worked. Taylor would then present the urine to the collector as his own. The rules were clear: The first positive was just a warning. The second was a four-game suspension. The third was a lifetime suspension with a possibility of being reinstated after one year, if the player followed league guidelines. Did Taylor's teammate feel guilty that his actions allowed L.T. to keep doing drugs without worrying about getting caught and suspended? "Not at all," he said. "He was a friend of mine and I was young. I wanted to win. I'm not saying I feel good about it."

The Giants' attempt to monitor and control drug use prior to 1987 was primitive. They left it up to Parcells. "Bill has always addressed the drug problem," Young said before Super Bowl XXI. "He recognized it as a problem and he's doing an excellent job. He's the one to discipline players and go face-to-face with them."

Parcells knew he had drug issues among the Giants besides Taylor. Prior to the league instituting its own testing program in the season after the Giants' first Super Bowl, Parcells conducted random tests on players he suspected were using drugs. He enlisted the help of the Giants training staff to handle the testing. He was not only fighting for his job in the early years; he was fighting to prevent a drug culture from bringing down his team. Parcells didn't worry about breaking rules by testing his players because there were no rules before 1987. In fact, even when there were rules in 1997 against teams conducting their own tests, Parcells was still aggressively drug testing at least one draft-eligible player on a visit to Weeb Ewbank Hall at the Jets facility at Hofstra University in Hempstead, New York. He had doubts about the player's character and passed on him. He was a high draft pick by another team and was out of the league seven years later following multiple suspensions and violating the league's drug policy seven times.

The Giants players knew that the only person who could stop Lawrence Taylor was L.T. They were wary of his mood swings and addiction to cocaine. Proving he was indeed Superman, Taylor walked out of rehab in 1986 and walked into the season and earned the MVP award, won the Super Bowl XXI title, and registered a career high in sacks. Taylor had an amazing ability to party during the week and dominate on Sundays.

The Giants had renewed Super Bowl aspirations in 1988. It was going to be a do-over after they were cheated in '87. Big Blue still had the foundation of their title team: Taylor, Simms, Banks, and Joe Morris, in addition to Carson and Martin, who planned to retire after the season. The Super Bowl coaching staff was largely intact as well.

Taylor had one positive test on his record from 1987, the first year the NFL tested. Whether he received the dirty urine from a teammate or produced it on his own, he lost all benefit of the doubt in the NFL's drug system. The breaking news flash came seven days before the opener against Washington: Taylor tested positive for cocaine for the second time, which brought a four-game suspension to start the season. It sent tremors through the locker room.

"We knew his lifestyle," Banks said. "I remember being deeply hurt when he was suspended. I called Bill Belichick right after the news came out and I was just so disappointed. I was still naive and felt let down, not understanding that these are personal failures and that it's a demon he's fighting. I was still supportive of Lawrence and pissed that it happened, but not pissed at him. You know what I mean?"

Taylor has said he tested positive because he had presented a teammate's urine, which he didn't know was dirty, as his own. "That's bullshit," a teammate said. "Lawrence bragged in his book [in 1987] about using urine of teammates and when he was tested in 1988, they were watching him. They made him pee in front of them."

Martin, one of the team leaders, tried to counsel Taylor many times before the suspension to try to help him get his life straightened out. He has a calm demeanor and a reassuring voice, but he was talking to an addict. "You see a guy who is self-destructing, you're not just going to buy a ticket and sit at ringside and watch it happen," Martin said.

It did no good.

Taking away a suspended player's game check can be a deterrent, but for Taylor, Sundays in the fall, taking him off the field is what cut the deepest. After getting the news he could not be around the team for a month, Martin told Parcells he was going to Taylor's house to make a wellness check.

"He needs someone," Martin said.

"George, don't go by there," Parcells said.

Parcells wanted things to settle down before anybody from the team, including him, intervened with Taylor. Parcells could always count on Martin to be a good soldier, but not this time. "I totally dismissed his advice," Martin said. "I had a colleague, a very dear friend, who was hurting, who needed someone."

Martin drove the thirty minutes from Giants Stadium to Taylor's house. He knocked on the door and Taylor's wife Linda appeared. Behind her was Taylor, who instead of getting ready for the season opener, was in his home, looking like a lost soul.

"Lawrence was down on the floor crying," Martin said. "What I saw was a broken man, a completely broken man. You see this guy who was a monster on the field, probably the greatest defensive player in the NFL, and he's on the floor crying. I was heartbroken. Linda was so appreciative that someone had come by and interceded and was at least showing some support to a man who had really toppled from the highest mountaintop. I met with Lawrence, and we had a very, very engaging episode. I didn't do anything other than say, 'I'm with you, there are a lot of guys who feel the same way, and you'll get through this.' That, in and of itself, is sometimes the greatest medicine that you can provide in a situation like that."

In a few months, Martin would be playing his final game in the NFL, and his compassion for his disgraced teammate sticks in his mind as one of the many life lessons learned. "I had seen him do things on the field that were inhuman, and I thought he had an air of invincibility," he said. "When I saw him in that very critical and vulnerable state, it spoke volumes to me that despite it all, we're human."

Carson didn't need the high from cocaine and didn't need drugs to be great. His father was an alcoholic, and Harry didn't drink and never went near drugs. Besides, he was team captain and felt obligated to set the right example for his teammates.

After the Giants played their final preseason game in 1988, they were given a few days off before preparation would begin for the season opener at home against Washington. Carson took advantage and went back home to South Carolina to visit his family. He had already announced he was retiring after the season, and George Young had already turned down his request for a raise, so when his sister gave him the message that Parcells was calling for him, he thought he was about to get cut.

"I'm very disappointed in you," Parcells said.

Carson laughed.

"Disappointed in what?" he said.

"You tested positive," Parcells said.

"Positive for what?" Carson said.

"Cocaine," Parcells said.

Parcells explained to Carson that when he got back to New Jersey he would have to submit to random drug testing by the league for the entire season. The closest Carson had ever come to cocaine was having Taylor as his training camp roommate at Fairleigh Dickinson University that summer. He met with his agent Craig Kelly at an attorney's office in New York to strategize how to challenge the test. Carson was furious but knew if he boycotted the testing, it would count as another positive test and would result in a four-game suspension. By not protesting, Carson was forced to submit to the dehumanizing procedure of having the collector watch him urinate, but with no suspension, the news did not go public. The New York newspapers never found out about Carson's positive test.

"Ask any one of my teammates who was the least likely to be involved in drugs, they would say Harry Carson," he said. "To have to deal with false accusations is something I've had to live with the rest of my life. To go through the indignity of peeing in a cup with somebody watching takes away your humanity."

Carson is convinced his urine was mismarked or switched when he submitted the standard training camp test in July. The league's urine collector took all the samples outside the dorms at FDU.

"I peed in a cup and moved on," Carson said. "I'm not on anything."

He had no reason to believe he would be peeing in a cup all season until speaking to Parcells. He felt betrayed by the Giants for not backing him up.

"Parcells, George Young, nobody believed me except [Giants team] Dr. [Russell] Warren when I said I didn't use drugs," Carson said. "I felt disrespected. I was pissed. I think that played a significant factor in my relationship with the Giants organization. Just the mere fact that I was their captain and nobody believed me—it was hurtful."

If his sample was intentionally switched rather than being an honest mistake, who would have done that? Carson suspects somebody in the Giants organization who didn't like him was out to get him. He never for a second suspected Taylor switching the cups. Besides, he tested positive also. "The mere fact that Lawrence and I were suitemates, I think most people would say, 'Well, you got two black guys, linebackers, one has a drug history, they're probably doing it together,'" Carson said. "For somebody who doesn't know I don't go near any kind of drugs to think this, it was painful for me."

All season, Carson walked down the corridor from the Giants locker room to the visitors' locker room at Giants Stadium and peed in a cup with the collector closely watching. The players' names were on the cups in plain view, making it impossible to be a confidential process, as the NFL promised. "The names are on the piss," Carson said. "So, I'm seeing who else is being tested."

Anybody being tested could also see that Carson was in the drug program. The entire experience left him looking forward to the end of the season and walking away from the NFL. But it wasn't the only time in his final year he was turned off by the organization not having his back. In the second week of November in a road game in Arizona, he had a loose chip floating in his knee that lodged in a joint. He needed arthroscopic surgery at the Hospital for Special Surgery in Manhattan. Doctors told him he should be back on the field in two weeks. As soon as he came out of the operating room, he was walking. The next morning, a Saturday, he was watching the news and was shocked to find out Parcells had put him on four-week injured reserve.

"I'm pissed about that," he said. "I felt Parcells lied to me."

It meant he would miss his final home game in Giants Stadium. Even so, the Giants honored Carson and George Martin before the game by acknowledging they were retiring after the season. Carson was still on IR and not in uniform. "There was a lot of tension going on there," he said. The next week, Carson returned, and the Giants lost to the Jets at Giants Stadium to knock them out of the playoffs. It was a Jets home game so his fans didn't get to see him play one last time.

"I ran off the field," Carson said.

He didn't stick around to shake hands or accept congratulations on a great career. "That was my last football game and I never looked back," he said. "I couldn't wait to get out of there. I was bitter."

His former coach with the Giants, John McVay, was the GM in San Francisco. McVay offered Carson more money than he was making with the Giants to play only as a first-down run stopper in 1989. The 49ers practices were well known by players around the NFL as the easiest in the league. Carson turned it down. He didn't want to wear another uniform. Then Parcells asked him to reconsider and play one more season because he didn't want to lose the leadership of Martin and Carson at the same time.

Shari, his wife at the time, was aware of the turmoil in his final season.

"Fuck Parcells," she said to Harry. "Fuck him."

The drug testing was conducted by the league, not the Giants. Asked about his feelings more than thirty years later about Carson testing positive for cocaine, Parcells said, "Harry didn't do drugs."

＝＝

THE GIANTS SPLIT their first four games of the 1988 season without Taylor and finished 10–6 and missed the playoffs by losing on tiebreakers to the Eagles for the NFC East title and the Rams for the NFC's second wild-card spot. Could Taylor have helped them beat Washington or San Francisco in the first four weeks? Of course. He returned for the final twelve games and had 15.5 sacks, the second-highest total of his career, and was voted first-team All-Pro. The Giants lost to the Jets 27–21 in the final game on Al Toon's touchdown catch with thirty-seven seconds remaining, eliminating them from making the playoffs.

The Eagles won the NFC East, led by defensive end Reggie White. He was an ordained minister at the age of seventeen and played the game drug-free, and he is a Hall of Famer and one of the most feared defensive players in NFL history. He did not party every night until the sun came up. He was not an addict. Even though White had those lifestyle advantages, Taylor was a better player. White took care of his body and had a longer career, but even with his clean living, he sadly died from heart issues and obstructive sleep apnea in 2004 when he was only forty-three years old. Taylor abused his body but has not experienced any serious health issues into his sixties.

If Parcells had his way, Taylor and White would have played together on the Giants. In the 1984 USFL supplemental draft, Parcells begged Young to take White with the third pick. The NFL was making contingency plans for distribution of USFL players with the expectation the league would eventually fold, which it did in the summer of 1986. Instead of taking White as Parcells preferred, Young drafted offensive tackle Gary Zimmerman, and the Eagles took White with the next pick. Zimmerman went on to be a Hall of Fame player, but not for the Giants. He refused to play in New York and was traded to the Vikings for two second-round picks, which Young turned into Collins, one of the best corners in Giants history, and safety Greg Lasker. Zimmerman won a Super Bowl with Denver in his final season in 1997.

Parcells and Belichick devising pass rush schemes for Taylor on the right side of the defense and White on the left side would have put together two of the great defensive minds and two of the great defensive players on one team. "With those two, our defense would have been illegal for a period of time," Parcells said. Belichick has called Taylor the best defensive player in NFL history. Taylor, in a rare moment of humility, lists White and Deacon Jones ahead of him. Either way, Taylor and White would have been incredible together. Young should have listened to Parcells.

Even more important, White was so respected and had such a strong personality he might have been a positive influence on Taylor's life if they had shared the same locker room. Regardless of Taylor's Monday through Saturday lifestyle, his coaches and teammates were unanimous: Taylor played his ass off on Sunday. He even played gunner on Belichick's punt coverage teams early in his career. He also played hurt: he put on a performance for the ages in 1988 in New Orleans late in the season of his drug suspension. The Giants were already without Simms, Banks, and Carson, but Taylor played with torn shoulder ligaments and detached pectoral muscle and a restrictive shoulder harness to keep everything in place. All he did was play in extraordinary pain and register three sacks, seven tackles, and two forced fumbles in an important 13–12 victory over the Saints.

"You were great tonight," Parcells told him in the locker room.

"I don't know how I made it," Taylor said.

He later said, "I wanted to cry because I felt like somebody had torn my shoulder off."

Banks was an impact player, but his accomplishments were overshadowed playing with Taylor and Carson, and that has cost him a spot in the Hall of Fame. Parcells and Belichick loved Banks, but nobody was a bigger fan than Taylor, who despite all his problems, was a great teammate. "If I got his stamp of approval, I don't think I need someone else's approval to say how good I was. Right? That's where I stand on that," Banks said. "You can say what you want. But this dude right here can tell you differently. And he can tell you why. And knowing that I could play at that level consistently was the biggest stamp of approval."

He does not resent that Taylor received all the publicity and all the credit. He was watching film with Taylor his rookie season in 1984. Banks made a play that caused Taylor to sit up in his seat. "That was a helluva play, homeboy," Taylor said.

When Banks heard that, he knew he had earned his respect.

There was a keepsake moment for Banks on the first play of the Giants playoff victory in '84 over the Rams in Anaheim. "Bill Parcells put a bounty out on Eric Dickerson," Banks said. "And he said he's got one thousand bucks for the first person who put Dickerson on his ass. So, the first play of the game, they ran it at me."

Rams quarterback Jeff Kemp pitched the ball to Dickerson, who had set an NFL record with 2,105 yards rushing during the regular season in just his second year in the league. Banks penetrated into the backfield and threw Dickerson for a four-yard loss. "And if you look at that clip, the guy who sprinted over to me, and jumped on me, was L.T.," Banks said. "He couldn't have been happier. So that's how that works out."

Taylor and Burt loved to compete with each other, especially on the golf course, and several times it nearly came to blows. If that ever were to happen, Taylor would be the stylish Muhammad Ali and Burt would be a bulldozer like Joe Frazier. It would be a helluva fight.

"I had a love-hate relationship with him. I'm not letting him get away with anything because he's Lawrence Taylor," he said. "That didn't mean shit to me."

Burt, Taylor, and Simms were playing in a charity golf tournament at Pine Valley Country Club, an exclusive club in southern New Jersey, where along with some members of the Giants front office, they were going to play with club members.

"I'll drive," Simms said.

"No. I'm going to drive," Taylor said.

Taylor got into the driver's seat of his new BMW 740. Burt and Simms knew Taylor's heavy foot on the highway, and they argued about who was sitting where. Neither wanted to sit in the front with Taylor. Burt won. He sat in the back.

"So, we're flying down the turnpike. Lawrence is speeding," Simms said.

"He was going 80 miles per hour," Burt said.

"I'm like, holy shit, slow down," Simms said.

A highway police officer gets even with Taylor and shouts on his speaker.

"Hey, slow it down!"

Taylor shrugged it off, and, as soon the cop drove off, he was back racing in the Jersey Turnpike 500. Simms said Taylor was dipping Skoal and spitting into a cup. He opened the driver's side window and tossed the cup onto the highway.

"When he rolled down the window, his ring went with it," Simms said.

At least it was not his Super Bowl ring.

"I don't want it anyway," Taylor said.

He kept driving.

"That dude was a wild cat, man," Burt said.

"It was scary the whole ride. I'm sitting there thinking I'm going to die," Simms said.

Taylor and Burt were paired on the golf course, which is always dangerous for the health of the fairway grass and the caddies. Simms knew from playing with them that this was not a good idea. "They are so competitive. I'm sure they were arguing the whole way around the course. And the course is hard," Simms said.

Simms's group finished first. When Taylor and Burt reached the eighteenth green, Simms asked their caddie how the round was going, knowing they gambled and argued about the rules. "Well, L.T. and Mr. Burt are having some words," the caddie said.

Simms and Burt found another ride home.

———

PARCELLS AND TAYLOR had a special relationship in the ten years they were together with the Giants, the last eight with Parcells as the head coach and the first two when he was defensive coordinator. "I just liked the idea that he actually knew who ran that team. I ran that team," Taylor said, laughing.

"Fucking Taylor," Parcells said. "I had fights with him that I'm not talking to the son of a bitch for three weeks. Sunday at one o'clock, you know where he is? Standing right next to me for the national anthem. That means, 'Parcells, you're an asshole, but I'm with you right now.'"

Parcells was accused of being Taylor's number-one enabler, a coach who needed to win to keep his job and was more concerned about keeping his best player on the field than getting him the help he required for his drug problems. Parcells says he tried to help Taylor more than anybody will ever know. "I worried about him a lot. Of course I did. He knows that," Parcells said. "What really stings my ass is when people say Parcells looked the other way. That is so much bullshit. There's not a fragment of truth to that. Not a shred. I didn't look the other way."

Two years after Taylor arrived, the Giants drafted LSU tight end Malcolm Scott in the fifth round. Parcells really liked him as a player and said he and undrafted rookie free agent Zeke Mowatt were both better than Jamie Williams, who was drafted in the third round. Williams played twelve years in the NFL, but none for the Giants. Mowatt played nine years, the first seven for the Giants, one for New England, before finishing up with one year back with the Giants. Scott played only one year for the Giants as a rookie in 1983 and three games for the Saints strike replacement team in 1987.

Drugs ruined Scott's career despite Parcells's effort to save him.

"Malcolm, he just got on that crack," he said. "So, I put him down in Fair Oaks. I get weights down to him so he can train while he's in rehab. I do everything to try to get him ready. Bring him back to camp. Finally, one night in camp he goes off the reservation. So, fuck it. I get rid of him. After Malcolm comes in, I said, 'Look son, I got to let you go. I can't do this anymore.' You know, he says to me, 'Coach, I'm sorry, you did everything you could, but it's just got me right now.' That was his answer. I said, 'Well, I hope you save yourself.'"

Quarterback Tommy Hodson, who played with Scott at LSU, was in New England for Parcells's first training camp as head coach of the

Patriots in 1993. Parcells asked him about Scott, and the answer was not good. Hodson told him that Scott was "fucking around hanging around Baton Rouge, he's not doing any good." Years later, Parcells heard that Scott had his own church in Atlanta and had become a preacher.

Parcells sent players to a drug counselor in Englewood, New Jersey. "Jane Jones," Parcells said. "I relied on her. She would tell me what the issue was. And then she would tell me how to treat them. Her best line was, 'Bill, you got to bust their balls. You threaten everything they got. You're trying to help, but if you can't help, here are the consequences.' We saved quite a few. Not all."

Taylor was the best player on the Giants. But he was not spared from Parcells diving deep into motivational tricks to get him fired up to face certain opponents. For the older players, he would leave gas cans in their lockers, the implication being: Do you have anything left in the tank? He left mouse traps in lockers after a big win preceding an easy opponent, the message intended to remind players not to let it be a trap game.

He once left a plane ticket to New Orleans on L.T.'s locker room stool a few days before a playoff game with the Rams in 1989. Taylor had trouble with Rams tackle Irv Pankey—he held Taylor without a sack earlier that season when L.T. had a sprained ankle. Yet Saints linebacker Pat Swilling had his way with Pankey. To light a fire under Taylor's ass, Parcells told him to fly to New Orleans and swap No. 56 jerseys with Swilling and send him to New York to face Pankey in the playoff game.

"If you wanted Pat Swilling, why didn't you draft the son of a bitch?" Taylor barked.

Result: Taylor beat Pankey for two sacks. The Giants lost anyway on Flipper Anderson's walk-off touchdown in overtime.

"Parcells, you know he has his way of coaching that maybe not a lot of players can handle," Taylor said. "But the guy, he's a winner, he loves to win. He turns over every stone and whatever it takes to get you fired up and ready for a game. At least for me, I mean, I don't need all that talking to and all that."

Parcells had a different relationship with Taylor than with any other player. He would get on Simms so hard in practice for every little mistake that Simms was unnerved by the time he walked in the door for dinner. Parcells relied on the wisdom of Carson and Martin. But with Taylor he had not only the perfect player with the perfect skills to coach, competitively Parcells found his match and knew the more he challenged him by appealing to his pride, the better he would play.

Neither could live with losing. Parcells tried to will his team to victory during the week. Taylor took over on Sundays.

"He wasn't just my coach. He was one of my best friends. He was my best friend," Taylor said.

"His relationship with Bill was truly incredible," Simms said. "Lawrence was a great player, one of the greatest that's ever played. And Bill could talk to him like nobody else. Bill could treat him just like any player on the team. And I think that's maybe why people didn't complain. Because he would get on Lawrence. There was just a small group that he would get on. And Lawrence was one of them. And I think it was really important. I didn't know that at the time. When you're playing you don't know much. You're just trying to do your thing. But yeah, Lawrence is one of those guys that he would call him out in practice, say things in front of other players, in front of the team. I think that was really good for everybody, it was good for Lawrence. It was good for our football team, for sure. And it just validated Bill Parcells even more in people's eyes."

Tom Brady never considered Belichick his best friend. Joe Montana and Bill Walsh were not best friends. Peyton Manning was closer to his offensive coordinator or quarterbacks coach than any head coach he played for in the NFL. Parcells would have done anything to keep Taylor away from drugs. The education and resources available then were not the same as they are today. Could he have done more? More can always be done.

"Bill has always been there for me. I've had problems, even out-side of football life," Taylor said. "I know I can always count on him. There's not a lot of guys you can count on, but there's some guys you can count on. Parcells was definitely one. Literally during those years, he was my best friend. Bill made it easy for me."

That was the foundation of the brotherhood. Always trying to help each other.

It was the ride of Bill Parcells's life. It doesn't get any better for a coach than to be carried off the field by his players, especially for Parcells, who grew up in New Jersey rooting for the Giants. He's a Hall of Fame coach who was skilled at knowing which buttons to push to get the most out of his players.

John Iacono/Getty Images

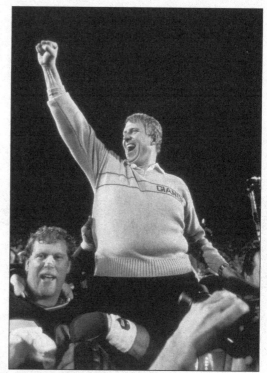

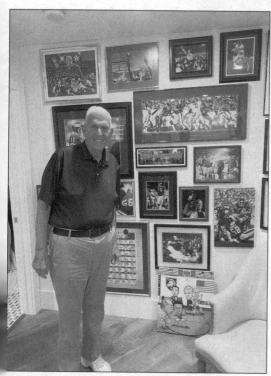

Bill Parcells's office right off the garage of his winter home in Tequesta, Florida, is filled with pictures honoring the "Parcells Guys" who helped him win two Super Bowls. His relentless style of coaching was not for everyone, but today he's the proud patriarch of the Super Bowl XXI championship team.

Gary Myers

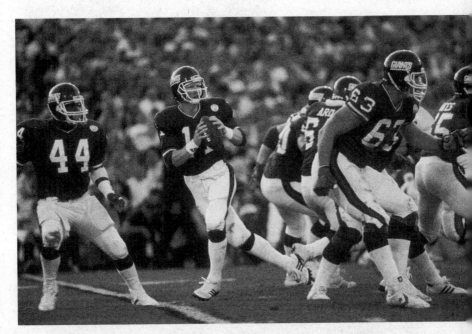

Phil Simms was on fire in Super Bowl XXI. He's the most underappreciated quarterback of the Super Bowl era. His 88 percent completions on twenty-two of twenty-five passes remains a Super Bowl record, and he will always be known as the first Super Bowl MVP to do the iconic "I'm going to Disney World" commercial.

Rob Brown/Getty Images

For two nights in a row after contracting COVID in the spring of 2021, Mark Bavaro fainted in his house. He had a pair of black eyes that made it seem like he put on eye black for a sunny afternoon game, but it was the darkest time of his life.

Courtesy of Mark Bavaro

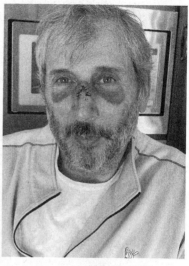

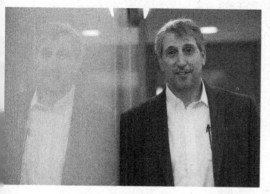

Mark Bavaro was so reluctant to speak with the media in his playing days that when one of his kids saw an interview he did in 1986, she scolded him, "Dad, you didn't know how to talk." His toughness and rugged looks made him a cult figure among Giants fans. Now he's as personable and talkative as any of the '86 Giants. *Susan Watts/New York Daily News*

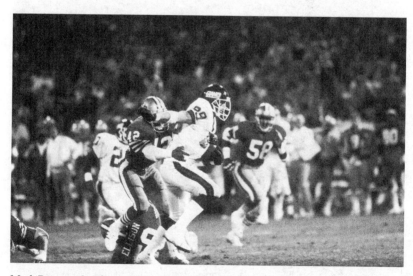

Mark Bavaro takes future Hall of Famer Ronnie Lott along for the ride, dragging and splattering half the 49ers defense on the way to an inspirational 31-yard gain in the third quarter of a 1986 late season Monday night game in San Francisco. It jumpstarted the Giants comeback from a 17–0 halftime deficit to beat the Niners 20–17 at Candlestick Park. *Jerry Pinkus/New York Giants*

Life after football has been a struggle for Bobby Johnson. A crack addiction led to him selling his Super Bowl ring for peanuts; suffering an accident in a pencil manufacturing plant that cost him half of his middle, ring, and pinkie fingers on his right hand;

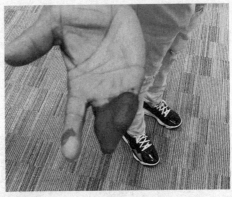

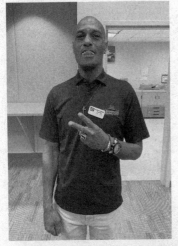

and living homeless on a park bench in Nashville. He eventually stopped his drug use on his own without going to rehab, and Bill Parcells helped buy back his Super Bowl ring for $30,000.

Gary Myers

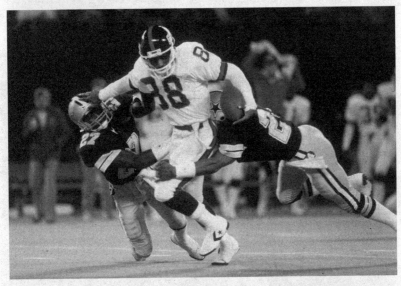

Phil Simms could always count on Bobby Johnson to catch anything he threw his way, as he did in this 1985 game at Giants Stadium against the Dallas Cowboys. The biggest play of his career came on his crucial first-down catch on fourth-and-17 in the final minute that led to the winning field goal in Minnesota in 1986. The victory convinced the Giants they could win the Super Bowl. *Jay Dickman/Getty Images*

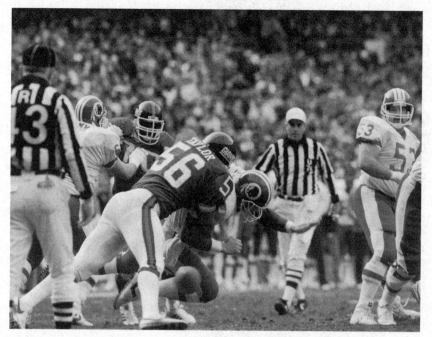

Two days before the Giants beat Washington in a crucial December game at RFK Stadium in '86, Lawrence Taylor was fast asleep under a chair in a defensive meeting. Awakened for a few minutes by an irritated assistant coach, he designed a new pass rush scheme and went back to sleep. Then he went out and sacked Washington quarterback Jay Schroeder three times. *Jerry Pinkus/New York Giants*

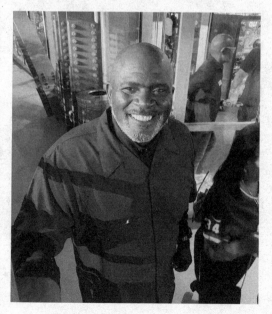

Lawrence Taylor insists "L. T.," his evil crack-addicted twin, the walking police blotter, is dead and buried, hopefully forever replaced by "Lawrence." When he returns to Giants games for a reunion, Taylor still receives the loudest ovation from fans, who always judged him on the field and not off it.

Gary Myers

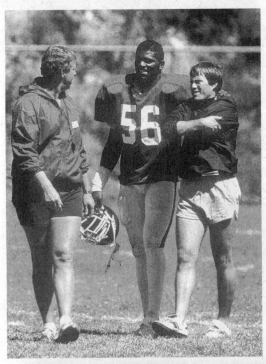

Bill Parcells, Lawrence Taylor, and Bill Belichick (*left to right*) get together at training camp in 1986 at Pace University in Pleasantville, New York. The greatest defensive player in NFL history and two of the greatest coaches helped put together a magical Super Bowl season. Taylor won the league's MVP award with a career-high 20.5 sacks.

Jerry Pinkus/New York Giants

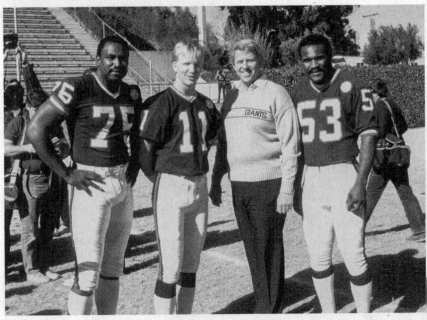

The inner circle of Bill Parcells was known as "Parcells Guys," the leaders he counted on to get his message across in the locker room. At the top of the list were the three captains in the Super Bowl XXI season: George Martin (75), Phil Simms (11), and Harry Carson (53). For the Super Bowl coin toss, Carson handled the responsibility by himself, surrounded by five Broncos. *Jerry Pinkus/New York Giants*

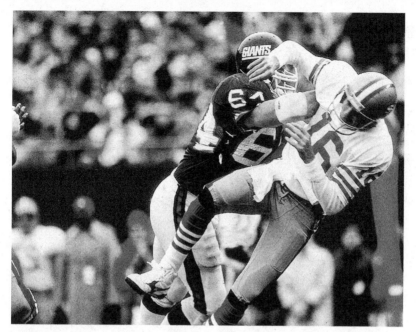

Every team needs a character to keep the locker room loose, especially after surviving one of Bill Parcells's grueling practices. Jim Burt was that guy for the Giants. In the divisional round of the 1986 playoffs in a 49–3 victory, he sent Joe Montana (his future teammate in San Francisco) in an ambulance to a Manhattan hospital with a crunching hit that resulted in a concussion. *Jerry Pinkus/New York Giants*

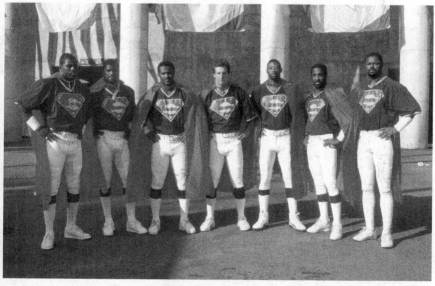

It's a bird, it's a plane . . . nah, it's just the Giants linebackers having some fun for charity the day before Super Bowl XXI. Gary Reasons rounded up the linebackers for a photo shoot at the Rose Bowl for a United Way poster. *From left to right*: Pepper Johnson, Lawrence Taylor, Harry Carson, Reasons, Carl Banks, Robbie Jones, and Andy Headen. *Jerry Pinkus/New York Giants*

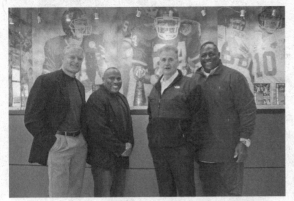

Bart Oates, Joe Morris, Jim Burt, and Leonard Marshall (*left to right*) reunited on a visit to the trophy case in the lobby of the Giants headquarters. All four of the team's Super Bowl trophies are on display, but it's the Lombardi Trophy from Super Bowl XXI, the team's first championship in thirty years visible between Morris and Burt, that represents the most beloved team in Giants history.

Robert Sabo/New York Daily News

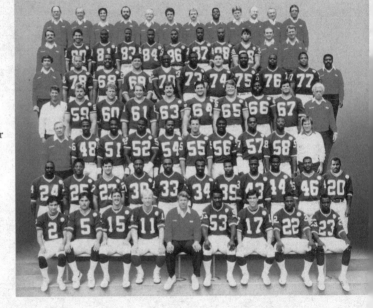

1986 New York Giants (see Appendix One for the 1986 Giants players' roster).

Jerry Pinkus/ New York Giants

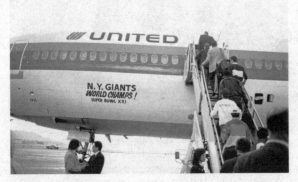

One day after the Giants demolished the Broncos in Super Bowl XXI, they walked onto the tarmac to discover a new design on the side of the team plane. That Tuesday they celebrated with fans at Giants Stadium after New York City mayor Ed Koch refused to pay for the traditional Canyon of Heroes ticker-tape parade because the team had moved to New Jersey ten years earlier.

Jerry Pinkus/New York Giants

PART II

WHAT IT TOOK TO WIN

4

BODY DOUBLE

Lawrence Taylor, Harry Carson, Bill Parcells, George Young, and the patriarch of the '86 Giants, Wellington Mara, have their busts displayed in the Pro Football Hall of Fame. Joining them in the Ring of Honor at MetLife Stadium from the '86 team are Phil Simms, Carl Banks, Mark Bavaro, George Martin, Leonard Marshall, Joe Morris, Ottis Anderson, and trainer Ronnie Barnes, who is so close to the Mara family that he's referred to as Wellington and Ann's twelfth child.

The Ring of Honor is an exclusive group selected by an internal committee led by team ownership. The names are displayed on blue banners on the facing of the stadium's upper deck at Giants home games. There are just fifty members covering the franchise's first ninety-eight seasons.

Membership in the Ring of Honor brings the players post-career visibility, creates opportunities in the business world, increases fees as a guest speaker, and gives access to the Giants forever. The players sign autographs with "Giants ROH" and the year they were inducted and jersey number. The collection from '86 comprises the elite of the best team ever from one of the NFL's historic and iconic franchises. The Ring of Honor guarantees their memory will be preserved long after they are gone.

Curtis McGriff is not in the ring. Maurice Carthon and William Roberts are not, either. Neither Gary Reasons nor Brad Benson have received the honor.

To win a Super Bowl, it's crucial to have Hall of Fame and Ring of Honor players, but it's also imperative to have players who are building blocks in the formative years and later become role players on a championship team. They pay the same physical price but without the glory and record-setting contracts.

McGriff was a building block deprived by injury of making it to Super Bowl XXI. Carthon and Roberts were role players who made it to the big game. They did not have the spotlight that followed Simms and Taylor, but all successful teams have selfless team-oriented productive players who help grind out victories. Benson was a cult hero because of a white bandage across the bridge of his nose that became the badge of honor of an overachieving true warrior. Even on a team dominated by stars in key positions, it takes players like McGriff, Carthon, Roberts, Reasons, Karl Nelson, Billy Ard, Chris Godfrey, and Benson to make a team complete.

McGriff played defensive end and won two national championships at the University of Alabama, including a famously clutch tackle at the goal line that helped topple top-ranked Penn State in the Sugar Bowl to win the title.

Even with his accomplishments in a championship program, McGriff was not picked in the twelve rounds of the 1980 NFL draft and signed with the Giants as a free agent. New York coach Ray Perkins had also played for Bear Bryant at Alabama and would later succeed him as the coach of the Crimson Tide. Perkins loved Alabama players. Bill Parcells arrived as the defensive coordinator in McGriff's second season, and the Giants switched from a 4-3 to a 3-4 defense with defensive end George Martin going from a three-down player to sharing the position with McGriff. Martin was the designated pass rusher; McGriff was the designated run stuffer.

"Curtis McGriff, that's my guy. I love that guy," Martin said. "Had it not been for Curtis, I wouldn't have played fourteen years in the

NFL because he took over the running responsibilities and I became a pass rushing specialist. Yeah, we are indebted to one another."

Martin is one of the most decorated players in Giants history. He was selected by Parcells to be his presenter at his Hall of Fame induction in 2013. Considering Parcells also coached Simms, Carson, Taylor, Curtis Martin, Ty Law, Tony Romo, and Demarcus Ware, it was a shock to George Martin.

"It's second only to winning the Super Bowl," he said. "When he asked me to do that, I thought he was joking. It was the greatest honor of my professional life."

Parcells first made the request in 2012, when new Hall of Fame rules put him on the ballot. Parcells had been a finalist for the Hall of Fame in 2001 and 2002 but failed to gain entry; voters were concerned he was not done coaching even though he claimed he had retired for good after stepping down with the Jets after the 1999 season. The voters were correct: Parcells was back in 2003 coaching the Cowboys. The Hall of Famer was later burned by Joe Gibbs, who retired from coaching Washington after the 1992 season, was elected in 1996, and came out of retirement to coach Washington from 2004 to 2007.

"George, if I'm inducted into the Hall of Fame, would you do me the honor of introducing me?" Parcells said.

Martin hesitated before answering.

"Come on, Bill, stop. Are you kidding?" Martin said.

"I'm totally serious," Parcells said.

Martin was featured on the video at Parcells's induction and walked on stage with him in Canton to remove the linen to reveal his bust. "To the outside viewer, it doesn't make any sense," Martin said. "Who the hell is George Martin compared to Lawrence Taylor, Harry Carson, Phil Simms, the guys on the Jets? Who was George Martin, compared to all the notable dignitaries in the National Football League and beyond, that could have had that honor? I don't know the answer. But I can tell you this: that just exudes the amount of respect and admiration that Bill and I had for one another."

McGriff was not in Bill Parcells's inner circle. But he was in George Martin's.

Martin was in his sixth season when McGriff was a rookie. McGriff's rookie salary in 1980 was $17,500. His game check after taxes was $900. When he began to chip away at Martin's playing time and eventually became the starter—run stoppers usually played first and second down in the '80s when the game was not as wide open as it is today—it provided an avenue for McGriff to increase his value and led to a larger contract. In his final year with the Giants in 1986, he made $180,000.

It came with a price for McGriff.

His health.

Playing the run in a 3-4 defense is more physical than any other position on the field. It guarantees multiple collisions every play. When the down marker flipped and it was an obvious passing situation, McGriff would run off the field, and Martin would take his spot on the left side of the defense. Run stoppers on a three-man line are blue collar and often double-teamed. Pass rushers get endorsements and commercials by playing a more glamorous role. Run stoppers were the equivalent of a stunt performer jumping off a cliff while George Clooney sits in a golf cart.

"Obviously, I was upset at not being the starter anymore," Martin said. "It was a mixed blessing."

Martin's job was to sack Roger Staubach, Joe Theismann, and Ron Jaworski. The game was more violent for McGriff. He was sticking his head in piles as a two-gap run stopper, trying to beat tackles and guards and get his arms around Tony Dorsett, John Riggins, and Wilbert Montgomery. He was responsible for the gap outside the right tackle and the gap between the right tackle and right guard. Martin just had to run straight ahead, put a move on a tackle, and hope to meet Taylor at the quarterback. He was not often double-teamed, with Taylor drawing most of the attention on the other side. Martin played at only 245 pounds, and the decision by Parcells to take him out of games on obvious running downs helped him extend his career and avoid the three dreaded letters: CTE.

The NFL was decades away from instituting a concussion protocol to not only protect players from overzealous coaches only worried about the game in front of them but also protect players from themselves.

Warriors play on until somebody tells them they can't. The NFL structure breeds job insecurity through its next-man-up mantra. Guaranteed money in contracts became common once free agency was introduced in the mid-'90s and relieved the pressure on the upper-middle and upper class to stay on the field or rush back sooner than their bodies were telling them. The fringe players barely making the league minimum still deal with that pressure.

McGriff knew he was doing a good job, but he also knew he was expendable if he was injured, or Parcells fell in love with a younger player. He was getting his "bell rung" more times than he can remember. "You bump heads every play," he said. "I probably had a concussion *every game*. You're bumping heads twenty to thirty plays a game—or more."

It was the Wild, Wild West in the '80s. Head trauma was not treated much differently than a sprained ankle. Rub some dirt on it and get back out there. Shake out the cobwebs. Players who got "dinged"—another code word for concussions—didn't sit the rest of the game, no less sit out the next game. "I had two diagnosed concussions," Martin said. "I was knocked silly against the Jets. I had to be helped to the sideline, was given smelling salts, and finished the game. Smelling salts was the cure-all. Two or three years later, I had another concussion on the kickoff team. Same thing. They waved smelling salts under my nose, and I got back in there. Nobody knew any better."

Carson estimates he had twelve to eighteen concussions playing football from high school on, most of them with the Giants either in practice or games. He retired after the 1988 season following thirteen seasons in New York and was diagnosed with post-concussion syndrome in 1990: headaches, blurred vision, sensitivity to light and noise, irritability, trouble retrieving words that used to be easy, spasms in his arm. He's better in his late sixties than he was in his mid-thirties. If he's in a particularly loud section of a restaurant with his wife, they switch tables. "You have to learn how to manage it," he said.

He is an outspoken advocate for players from previous generations who helped grow the league into the $18 billion a year industry it is today. He ad-libbed his Hall of Fame speech, concentrating on his plea to the NFL not to forget retired players who need help with health issues and medical expenses. Even with the added scrutiny brought by a class-action concussion lawsuit that required the NFL to reluctantly pay out $1 billion in concussion claims to former players, and with the implementation of rules to protect the quarterback and defenseless receivers, there isn't anything that can be done to prevent violent collisions like the trainwreck between Carson and Riggins, the Washington running back.

Sadly, it's these confrontations that make the NFL so popular and impossible for fans to turn away.

It was 1984. Giants at Washington. Riggins had the ball. Carson's job was to shed blockers and bring him down. The impact of two strong and highly competitive future Hall of Famers weighing a combined 467 pounds meeting helmet-to-helmet at the point of attack shook the foundation of old RFK Stadium.

"Power against power," Carson said. "It was like two trains, two diesel trains, hitting together. When we collided, everything faded to black for me."

He was proud to say, "I got up."

He was literally out on his feet.

Carson somehow stumbled back to the Giants huddle. "That was during the time we held hands in the huddle," he said. "I squeezed the guy's hand next to me. I thought I was going to go down."

But not out of the game.

He was the play caller on defense and looked to Bill Belichick on the sideline for what he wanted to run. Belichick used the customary hand signals in the pre–radio helmet days to get the defensive forma-tion to Carson. "I see Belichick—he flashed a signal, and I can't inter-pret what defense he wanted me to play," Carson said.

Carson stared at Belichick and tapped his helmet. "Meaning, I don't get it," he said.

That was the sign for Belichick to send him the call again.

"I still didn't comprehend what it was," he said.

Rookie Gary Reasons, playing inside linebacker next to Carson, covered for him and interpreted the signal from Belichick. "Gary saw it and Gary made the call," Carson said. "I stayed in and when the play was over everything was fine. You don't stop to think, 'Did I get concussed?'"

He was.

He didn't tell the trainers. He never self-reported after he got his "bell rung" or was "dinged."

"It was a whole different mind-set back then. I was about playing the game," he said.

Carson was an All-Pro and had as much job security as any player on the Giants, even in 1984, his ninth year in the league. The NFL dis-posed of players once the tread on their tires wore a little thin, but Carson was still playing at a high level. Whether he irrationally feared for his job, felt an obligation to stay on the field for his teammates, or reveled in his battlefield mentality, he didn't do the right thing for his long-term health.

Where was Parcells when his players were getting concussed? "We had the team doctors. They were the ones looking at the guys," Parcells said. "The whole process was vastly different than it is today. There wasn't a protocol."

But there was common sense. If the majority of players didn't have it, then it was incumbent upon the coaches and doctors to pro-tect the players. Carson and Parcells are correct. It was a different era then. Not nearly as much was known about concussions. Allowing a player who was seeing stars—and it was not difficult to identify those out on their feet—to remain on the field was wrong in any era. The attitude through the early part of the 2000s was the first concussion did not make a player immediately more susceptible to a second. Nobody spoke about the brain needing a chance to heal.

Players who came off the field woozy and drew the attention of the medical staff on the sidelines didn't have to pass tests given by an independent neurologist. All they basically had to do was count to ten; say their name, the day of the week, and what stadium they were playing in; take a whiff of smelling salts, and off they went back into the game. One Giants player once was encouraged to return to the game because his team needed him although he clearly had suffered a concussion a few minutes earlier and was surrounded by the medical staff. The player went in for the next series, the Giants scored, and he returned to the bench. Before the game was over, he got up and attempted to walk toward the locker room at Giants Stadium but became disoriented and went into the wrong tunnel. One of the coaches saw that the player was lost and sent a member of the support staff to retrieve him and walk him to the locker room.

McGriff's motive for staying in games after he had his bell rung, was dinged or concussed, was simple: He liked his job and wanted to keep it. He knew Parcells could replace him at any moment of any game. His job security went play to play, week to week.

"Shit, when you're the walk-on free agent, you ain't going to tell the coach you can't go play," he said. "Shit, I wouldn't want to tell them I couldn't do it because guess what: Next man up. Go get the next flight out of town. Hell, no."

McGriff played in all thirty-two regular season games, starting thirty, in the two seasons leading up to the Super Bowl. But he missed the entire 1986 season after suffering a hamstring injury in a preseason game against the Packers at Milwaukee County Stadium on August 16 and was placed on season-ending injured reserve.

That was not good news for Martin. He started only thirteen games in the previous five seasons, but without McGriff to play his body double on running downs, he was forced to return to his previous role as a full-time player in '86, starting all sixteen regular season games and all three playoff games, including the Super Bowl. It was no surprise that the full-time work reduced Martin's production at age thirty-three. He had only three sacks after recording ten sacks one year earlier as a part-time player. It was the fewest of his career other than his rookie year in 1975 when he started just three games and didn't record a sack. Martin's risk factor for injury went up without McGriff playing the more physical running downs. "It was uncomfortable at first," Martin said. "We had a real good supporting cast, but I sorely missed Curtis. We had a very good rotation. We were a tag team."

The Giants had just drafted defensive end Eric Dorsey from Notre Dame in the first round, nose tackle Erik Howard in the second round, and defensive end John Washington in the third, but none of the rookies were better options than Martin to take over for McGriff on a team deemed ready to make a long playoff run.

McGriff had done all the dirty work leading up to '86, but football is an unforgiving sport. He was a key contributor in the buildup to the Super Bowl season but lost out on the thrill of being on the field with his teammates during their magical ride. He didn't know it at the time, but he would never again play in a regular season game for the Giants. They waived him in the final cutdown one week before the opener in 1987 and replaced him with Dorsey. He gave his body to the Giants, was very good at one of the toughest jobs, but was dumped as soon as Parcells decided the needle on his tank was trending toward empty.

Next man up.

McGriff played just one more game in his career when he signed as a replacement player for Washington during the 1987 strike. He did not register any defensive statistics in Washington's 38–12 victory over the Giants' replacement players and was not retained after the twenty-four-day strike ended.

It's easy to forget McGriff's impact on a star-studded defense, but he set the standard for a two-gap defensive end in Parcells's scheme. Hall of Fame offensive tackle Jackie Slater, in a *Sports Illustrated* story, recalling the top players he faced, noted "an old widebody from the Giants, a guy you just couldn't block out of a play. Curtis McGriff."

THE POWER CORNER in the Giants locker room was right by the entrance a few steps from the players' lounge with a television and pay phone. Carson was closest to the door, then Taylor and Martin. Belichick said in *A Football Life* that when defensive line coach Romeo Crennel's daughter was commissioned to clean up Taylor's messy locker, she found $75,000 in uncashed checks.

Carson and Martin were the longest-tenured Giants on the '86 team. They were from South Carolina and experienced racism growing up. "I was never threatened with violence," Carson said. He remembers the Ku Klux Klan driving through the Black neighborhoods of his hometown of Florence with their horns blasting and hearing them say, "Go back to where you came from." His schools didn't become integrated until the eleventh grade. Until then, he had never gone to school with a white classmate.

Martin survived even worse. He lived in Greenville until the sixth grade before his father, who was in civil service in the military, was transferred to Savannah, Georgia. "I was a country boy living in the segregated South," he said. "I lived in Greenville long enough to know that I never would go back there and make it home. I can tell you that."

He dispassionately rattled off the atrocities. "Pick a day. Being threatened to be lynched, being called a nigger every other day. Being threatened as a young kid by adults, that you can't go in here and you can't drink over there. That you can't look at a white woman or otherwise you'll get beat up, you'll get killed, you'll be lynched," he said. "America has come a long way. I'm so fortunate and grateful that was something I was able to overcome."

Martin has enjoyed a successful post-football life. He's had no memory loss issues, other than the normal lapses accompanying the aging process. He's physically fit, which he displayed walking across the country, starting at the George Washington Bridge on September 16, 2007, and ending in San Diego on June 21, 2008, to raise money and awareness for rescue and recovery workers suffering respiratory problems after 9/11. He walked 3,003 miles, went through twenty-four pairs of shoes, eighty pairs of socks, lost forty pounds, and raised over $2 million. He still walks six and a half miles every other day, works out in the gym, and schedules regular doctor's visits.

"I cherish the fact that I can still walk and speak and talk intelligently," Martin said. "I've had no ill effects from football. My health today is spectacular. I've always approached myself as realizing that I had a life after football. And I always said this, when I played, that I want to be able to pick up my grandkids and hug them and be able to interact with them when I get to a certain age. I have six grandkids. I take them fishing, I hike with them, I pick them up, I put them on my shoulders. That's not to say that, yeah, fourteen years as a defensive lineman, you come away totally unscathed. You know, there's a shoulder injury, a knee injury, a hip injury, that are going to come with age anyway."

McGriff's presence helped lead to a healthier life after football for Martin, even if his stand-in has not been so fortunate mentally, physically, or financially.

Martin was vice president of human resources in New York for Tanagraphics, the third-largest printing company in the United States. In the early '90s, "Curtis was looking for employment," Martin said. "I went to ownership and asked if they could give him a position."

McGriff was hired as a security guard. He did well enough that he was given a promotion. There was a *New York Times* story in 1987 reporting that McGriff sold his Super Bowl ring. "Not true," he said. "I'm wearing it right now." Twenty years after his football career ended, McGriff took a job as a teacher's assistant at the High Point School of Bergen County, an alternative school of thirty to fifty at-risk students from eighth through twelfth grade in Lodi, New Jersey. McGriff said many of the students had been expelled from schools in Paterson, Jersey City, and Newark.

The school's mission statement of its behavior modification program reads:

The High Point behavioral program is an intensive, proven-effective behavior modification system designed specifically for students with significant and complex academic, behavioral, and social-emotional needs. This system is driven by the concept of positive reinforcement, informed by leading research in the fields of behavioral science and behavior modification, designed to minimize classroom disruptions and maximize learning time, and modeled and motivated by the students themselves.

In the fall of 2013, McGriff's wife noticed he was exhibiting behavioral changes. "She said I wasn't the guy she married," McGriff said. Over a six-month period into March, things did not get better. Mood swings, anger, memory issues. One day at school, he was informed one of his male students had wandered into another classroom. McGriff was told to bring him back, and the young man, about eighteen years old and, according to McGriff's description, "six foot and probably one hundred ten pounds," locked himself in the classroom.

"He was clowning like this was a joke," he said. "I told him, 'Dude, this ain't no joke, man.'"

McGriff could feel rage building inside. "I was going back to game day," he said. "My mind took me there."

The classroom was on the second floor.

"Curtis went berserk on some kid," Carson said. "He was thinking of throwing the kid out the window."

McGriff admitted he had to fight back the urge to toss the kid out the window. He had worked at the school for several years, but this was the first time he snapped. "Those bad things were going through my mind," he said. "All it took was me to do what my mind was saying, and it would have been a bad situation."

Thankfully, he said, he never placed his hands on the boy.

Instead, he walked into the school superintendent's office and resigned.

"Most of these kids come from bad backgrounds, and school is the only love they are getting," he said. "And if I can't give the kid the love that he is coming here for, I'm in the wrong business. It was time for me to get out of there and get help."

As most of the '86 Giants do when they have a problem, the first phone call went to Carson. McGriff told him about his anger and how he controlled himself to prevent a tragedy. Then he broke the news:

"He said he felt like he was suicidal," Carson said. "I said, 'Curtis, listen, whatever time you have these feelings, you have my permission to call me around the clock.' This was in the morning. He called me about two in the afternoon and said, 'Thanks, Harry. You saved my life.'"

His anger management issues had progressed prior to that day at school to the point that he feared if he went into a bar and somebody pissed him off by saying the wrong thing at the wrong time, his mind-set would shift and "go full speed," he said. He was no longer willing to take that risk.

McGriff didn't immediately recall his conversation about suicide with Carson until reminded. "I forget a lot. But if Harry said I said it, he's right. I was having some bad thoughts," he said. "You know what? I didn't give a damn if I lived or died." He pushed that to the side long enough to seek medical help. "I didn't control me getting here. I'm not going to control me leaving here. God can do all that," he's able to say now. "I don't care how bad it gets; I'm never going to intentionally do that. Something is wrong with me if I kill my damn self."

The event at the High Point School was the turning point in his adult life. He had been reading about CTE and the deaths by suicide of many former NFL players. He went to see a neurologist. "What he found was consistent with people in car crashes," McGriff said. "He mostly dealt with brain injuries and that kind of stuff. I had some of the same symptoms of people that have brain trauma."

The doctor found the right meds to get McGriff back on track. McGriff believes his mental health issues are related to all those collisions he had every game for six years with the Giants and his years playing at Alabama and in high school. "I didn't get this working nine-to-five on the assembly line," he said.

He and his wife decided to move back to Alabama. He collected money from the class action concussion lawsuit, and teammates say that helped him and his sister buy a house built in 1950 in Gordon, Alabama, on a twenty-four-acre piece of property. They remodeled it into CW's Country Living and Resort. His family still owns the hundred-acre property in Alabama that his grandfather bought in 1882. "I come from an era of picking cotton in the Deep South," he said. "We never did no sharecropping, but we lived off the land."

He is comfortable back home. He's had four operations, including surgery on his back and shoulder, since his playing days. He had two knee surgeries with the Giants. He said he can't remember what he had for lunch yesterday, but if he's asked a story about playing for Bryant, "I can reach back and grab that."

He operates a four-wheeler with his German shepherd riding shotgun to drive twice a week to the family farm with cows and hogs. When he goes out of town, it's never alone. "I got to have someone with me," he said. "Finding places, it's hard to do."

McGriff said he has no regrets about playing football. It took him from playing high school ball in Cottonwood, Alabama, to Tuscaloosa for big-time college football and on to New York, where he earned a Super Bowl ring. Football allowed his mother and father to travel to see him play and visit cities they otherwise never would have experienced.

"That made me feel good," he said. "The journey was worth it."

Martin makes sure he stays in touch with McGriff, knowing communication is the key to providing help to any teammate who needs it. "We all are in this sort of communication. We chime in about current events, and we just stay in contact to see how one another's doing," Martin said. "We are always looking over one another's shoulder because we don't want any of our inner circle to fall through the safety net or become indigent. So, we try to make sure that we have a nice communication."

CARSON TAKES HIS role as captain to heart. He has life experiences to pass on to teammates and relates to McGriff's suicidal thoughts because he had his own.

He became a father for the first time when his daughter Aja was born in 1979. He didn't have the nerve to tell his mother, Gladys. "Because I was a mama's boy, I was raised a certain way in the South. I thought my mother would be disappointed in me because I was having a baby out of wedlock," he said. "I was waiting for the right time to tell her. I didn't tell anybody in the family."

Gladys, who had an eighth-grade education, left her family behind in Florence when Carson was six years old to accept a job as a domestic worker in Newark, New Jersey. "It was her way of helping to support the family," Carson said. He lived with his father, his sisters, and his great aunt. He wrote letters to his mother constantly. Gladys had been working in the kitchen at the Florence Country Club and bringing home leftover food for Harry and his sisters. His father was laid off from his job with the railroad in South Carolina and found work driving a taxi. He was given rail passes as a former employee that allowed Carson to come north to visit his mother. "I was always her baby," Carson said. "Even when I was twenty-five years old, she'd still want me to sit on her lap." When the Giants drafted Carson in 1976, he was able to spend quality time with his mother, who was still in Newark. If the Giants were playing a home game at 4 p.m., he would take her to church in the morning. On days off, he would take her shopping at the mall in Paramus Park.

Harry convinced Gladys to leave Newark and move back to Florence once he was making good money after a few years with the Giants. He regrets never informing his mother about Aja before she was born. He never got the chance after she was born.

Carson was visiting his mother in Florence in her two-bedroom apartment during the third trimester of his girlfriend Ann's pregnancy in 1979. He and his brother Edgar went to her bedroom and found her unconscious. She had suffered an aneurysm. "The ambulance came, put her on a gurney and took her downstairs and to the hospital,"

Carson said. "She was in the local hospital, and there was nothing more they could do for her."

Doctors suggested moving Gladys to Duke University Medical Center in Durham, North Carolina, which was 175 miles away. Carson chartered a plane for her and then went back to New York to be with Ann, who was about to give birth. "I never had the opportunity to tell my mother she was going to be a grandmother," Carson said sadly.

Aja was born at 4:49 p.m. on June 2 by cesarean section. "I called and gave the news to my family," he said. Edgar went into their mother's hospital room and told her even though she was still not awake. "The only way that we know she knows is her vital signs kind of flickered," Carson said. Gladys never regained consciousness and died on June 16. "It was very difficult for me to accept," Carson said. "What I have come to accept is all the love that I had for my mother flowed over to Aja."

It was Aja's love that saved Carson from driving into the Hudson River.

Carson had an apartment in Ossining, New York, about an hour's drive up the Hudson River from New York City. After Aja was born, he moved with Ann and the baby to a bigger condo on Lincoln Place in the same town. As time went on, Carson and Ann were growing apart. He was educated. She was a high school dropout. He encouraged her to get her GED and helped her get into Pace University where the Giants held training camp. She wanted to become a nurse but dropped out after one semester. She drank too much. She smoked marijuana. Eventually, he said he found out she was doing crack. Carson never smoked weed or crack or snorted coke. One day he walked into his townhouse and she was getting high with a friend. Carson wrote Ann a note that he wanted custody. She moved to California, and he raised Aja as a single father.

She was daddy's little girl. Just as he was mama's little boy. Aja was his life. Carson was mother and father, doing her hair in the morning, reading bedtime stories, taking her to school and the Bronx Zoo, bringing her to training camp to show off to his teammates.

Carson never loved football. He found out in high school that putting on a football uniform was a "chick magnet," which helped draw him to the sport. "I look good in a uniform," he said. He doubled down on the uniform by joining ROTC—he came from a military family and had a genuine interest in becoming a fighter pilot. He rose to lieutenant colonel in the ROTC program at his high school. For a tough football player, he was a sensitive guy. After he played poorly in a Monday night game in Philadelphia in the third week of the 1980 season, he refused to accept his paycheck and told the Giants to donate it to charity and that he planned to retire immediately. News spread throughout the locker room and reached head coach Ray Perkins, who asked to meet with him in his office at the stadium the next day. Carson brought Aja with him. Perkins told him he needed him and talked him out of quitting. He played eight more seasons.

Before Carson moved to Washington Township in New Jersey in 1982, the Tappan Zee Bridge was the quickest way to get to Giants Stadium for workouts, practices, and games. Until the bridge was replaced in 2017 by the Mario Cuomo Bridge with high fences, the Tappan Zee was known as a jumper's bridge.

"I would occasionally go across the Tappan Zee and see where people would stop their car on the bridge and jump off," he said. "I never really thought about it. Then one day, I don't know, I was depressed about something. And I thought to myself, 'Maybe I should accelerate, go through the guardrail and just go over.' I'm thinking about this. I thought about it for a day or two. I thought to myself, 'What would happen to Aja?'"

He couldn't leave her. "That is why Aja was really my saving grace," he said.

Carson has spent years trying to dissect why he was having a mental health crisis. "I was playing ball, had a nice car, money. I wasn't hurting for anything. There were things that weren't necessarily golden at the time, but I couldn't figure out why I am depressed, but here I am thinking about ending my life," he said. "It was the thought of what would become of my daughter that really did play into my life at the time. I had a conversation with Aja not long ago and told her, 'You saved my life, if it had not been for you . . .'"

His voice trails off. "I've always been kind of impulsive," he said.

He's come to understand the concussions he suffered up to that point in his career could have been responsible for his depression and suicidal thoughts. CTE was just three letters in the alphabet that together didn't mean anything in the early '80s. In his final season in the NFL in 1988, Carson felt depression coming over him again. He went into the training room and told Barnes. "I'm probably the only person who put his name down listing depression on the injury report," he said.

Two years after Carson retired, he went for his annual physical and then two additional days of more intense testing. He was diagnosed with post-concussion syndrome. "I didn't know what that was," he said. "I thought, quite frankly, about Doug Kotar."

Kotar was a Giants running back from 1974 to 1981. He retired on the first day of training camp in 1982 because of knee and shoulder injuries. He was also suffering from terrible headaches, which he initially thought resulted from a kick in the head during a water volleyball game. Three weeks after retiring, Kotar was visiting the New York area and went for a CAT scan at the hospital at the University of Medicine and Dentistry of New Jersey in Newark. Tests revealed a tumor the size of a golf ball. It was malignant and doctors determined it was too risky to remove. He was transported to Presbyterian Hospital in Pittsburgh near his home to receive chemotherapy and radiation treatments. He died on December 16, 1983, just sixteen months after he was diagnosed. He was thirty-two years old.

"After they opened him up, they gave him six months to two years," Carson said. "I was thinking I had the same thing."

Carson asked his doctor if he was going to live. The doctor assured Carson he did not have a brain tumor and just had to learn how to manage headaches, light sensitivity, and irritability and not become frustrated if his memory failed him.

He thought back to the Tappan Zee Bridge. "I'm a happy-go-lucky guy," he said. "Just contemplating ending my life is heavy, you know?"

===

LEONARD MARSHALL WAS living in Hackensack, New Jersey, in 2010, in the Camelot apartment building on Prospect Avenue, having just moved back up north from Boca Raton, Florida, after the breakup of his marriage. The transition was made easier because former teammates Zeke Mowatt and McGriff also had apartments in the Camelot. He was going through a contentious divorce with "my dumb-ass ex," he said. They had a daughter together. He was annoyed with the lawyers and the inability to resolve things with his wife on their own. "All I really want out of this is for my daughter to know I'm not divorcing her. I'm divorcing myself from her mom," he said. "I couldn't seem to make heads or tails of that. And so that's what kind of drove me into darkness."

He had a lot of physical issues from playing football. He's convinced he has CTE and said he's been told he has early-stage Parkinson's. Head trauma from football left him with post-career headaches. By his count, he absorbed three hundred thousand hits to the head in his career between practices and games. He has ruptured discs in his neck and back. Football, he said without hesitation, caused physical and mental issues and destroyed his marriage. To help pay it forward, he has made arrangements to donate his brain after he dies to Boston University's Chronic Traumatic Encephalopathy Center.

He felt trapped in 2010. The divorce proceedings were dragging. As he stood in the kitchen of his girlfriend Lisa's apartment in North Arlington, he was ready to check out. He made a decision he doesn't regret. He dialed 911.

"I called the police department and said, 'I think I need help,'" Marshall said.

He was afraid in that moment of despair, just as Carson had experienced and McGriff would later experience, he was going to kill himself. "You never know to what extent a man could become that weak," he said. The police arrived at his house in a hurry. By then, his future wife Lisa had calmed him down. He told the police, "No, no, no. I'm not that weak, guys. I'm stronger than that. I'm tougher than that. I'll be fine."

He leaned on Carson and Martin. He relied on family. He became a proponent of CBD products that help with headaches. He married Lisa. He consulted with Bennet Omalu, the doctor who discovered CTE, portrayed by Will Smith in the movie *Concussion*. After living in a condo development where there was no privacy, he bought a big house with a lot of property and green grass and trees in Jackson Township, New Jersey.

"I have great days and days when it's a struggle," he said.

Marshall was inducted into the Giants Ring of Honor in 2022, recognition he thought was a long time coming. He's proud of his career and how he's dealing with life after football. He copes with the headaches and restricts light coming into his house by pulling down the shades.

During the years he lived in Boca Raton, every day was a challenge. He was behaving erratically, had a short fuse, and the light coming through his windows by his pool aggravated him. "There would be days where I get depressed as hell, you know, my mind would start working against me," he said. "I was wondering if other guys were dealing with the same shit, and then I start getting calls from them."

The easiest tasks became a struggle. Then he started to invent tasks. He was sitting in the Publix supermarket parking lot not only questioning what he needed but perplexed he was at the store in Deerfield Beach and not in Boca. He called his wife. She was confused why he was not at home.

"I thought you asked me to go to the store," he said.

"No," she said.

"I don't know why I am here," he said.

"Come on home," she said.

The fear of driving alone and getting lost is a common theme among the '86 Giants who suffered head trauma.

"When everybody chose to play football, they could clearly see getting hurt physically. You assume that risk," Carson said. "You can't blame anybody for the aches and pains. From a physical standpoint, you know you could get hurt. From a neurological standpoint, you did not know. Now the information is there."

Twenty years too late for the '86 Giants.

═══

MAURICE CARTHON WAS a throwback, a fullback who occasionally ran the ball but was on the roster primarily to block for a big-money tailback. Fullbacks have become all but extinct in the wide-open NFL, where the third receiver or second tight end are used instead to create a one-back backfield, which in Carthon's days was run by Washington with Riggins and few other teams.

Carthon was an unsung hero of the '86 Giants, creating space for Joe Morris in the running game and picking up blitzes in front of Simms in the passing game. He was one of Parcells's favorite players and was among the early arrivals in the locker room on game day, shooting the shit with his coach and holding court with a cup of coffee in his hand.

He felt appreciated by Parcells and the Giants. That was not the case in the USFL. He enjoyed his three years in the New Jersey Generals backfield with Herschel Walker but didn't have warm feelings about the Generals' owner, future president Donald Trump. Carthon played in all three of the USFL's seasons from 1983 to 1985, and it was during the third year that it became known that after the spring season finished, he would sign with the Giants before training camp. In what was a true test of his ironman skills, Carthon went from the USFL season to Giants training camp with just a couple of weeks off. Counting preseason, regular season, and playoff games, he played in forty-five football games in an eleven-month period. Trump kissed up to Walker and Doug Flutie, the main attractions of his team, and didn't value Carthon the same way. Carthon knew that when he bumped into Trump at a football luncheon. Trump, who bought the Generals after their first season, was not aware Carthon was leaving.

"I want you to know, people don't come to see you play. They come to see Herschel Walker and Doug Flutie," Trump said.

"Doesn't matter. I've signed with the Giants. They can come to see me play with them," Carthon said.

"Why don't you just call your agent? We'll get this done," Trump said.

"Too late," Carthon said.

The USFL never played another game. Trump's attempt to move the USFL season to the fall in 1986 to compete with the NFL failed miserably. He filed a $1.69 billion antitrust lawsuit against the NFL; his goal was for a settlement that would absorb the Generals into the NFL. Instead, the jury awarded the USFL just $1 in the summer of '86, which NFL lawyer Frank Rothman offered to pay out of his own pocket to USFL lawyer Harvey Myerson as they were walking out of Judge Peter Leisure's courtroom.

Trump was all but laughed out of the courthouse and onto Pearl Street in lower Manhattan. Carthon was already in his second Giants camp, having proved to be a seamless fit in the offense at the time the USFL closed down. He quickly became a locker room leader on a team already filled with leaders. Simms discovered that Carthon was the most honest person he knew: He would criticize teammates for not doing their job and call them out for not knowing their assignments. He kept teammates accountable. "He was incredible," Simms said.

Martin had Carthon and his wife over for Thanksgiving dinner in his first year with the Giants. They have remained friends and take part in a texting chain with eight other teammates. When Martin was doing his walk across America, his route took him through the Phoenix area when Carthon was the running backs coach for the Cardinals. Carthon made sure to see Martin when he stopped off in a park.

Carthon won the first of his two Super Bowl rings with the Giants in 1986. He later went on to coach for Parcells with the Patriots, Jets, and Cowboys, and interviewed for head coaching jobs with the Packers, Raiders, and Saints. He was a casualty of the NFL's poor record hiring minority head coaches. Carthon was an assistant coach on seven teams, and his last stop was Kansas City, where he worked on the staff of Chiefs head coach Romeo Crennel, the former Giants defensive line coach, who is also African American. Crennel and his assistants were fired after the 2012 season.

Carthon did not coach in 2013 and returned to his home in Jonesboro, Arkansas. He was sitting on his couch watching college football bowl games on January 1, 2014, with a police officer buddy. His post-football body was in good shape, relatively speaking. He needed to have a hip replaced. He suffered some memory loss, which was likely the result of being the lead blocker for Walker, Morris, and Ottis Anderson. High blood pressure was a trait in Carthon's family, but he had foolishly stopped taking his medication. His friend noticed Carthon didn't look good when they were watching the games.

"Maurice, you look like you've having a stroke," he said.

"No. You got to be kidding me," Carthon said.

"Let me do my job and get you to the hospital," the friend said.

They called Carthon's doctor, who advised them to get him on a helicopter to a hospital in Memphis fifty miles away. He was given what he called a "stroke pill" that saved his life. Another few minutes, and he would have been dead. He was just fifty-three years old.

His speech is now halting, and he takes long pauses before answering questions. He suffers from short-term memory loss. "I'm thinking clearly," he said. "At one time, speech-wise, I really couldn't talk after the stroke. It still bothers me a little bit to talk. Sometimes I talk too fast and will stutter. I've learned to try to control myself and not speak as fast. I find sometimes I get overwhelmed speaking too fast. I've come a long way."

He made two trips to Houston with his mother and sister relating to the concussion lawsuit. "They were talking about millions and millions. It wasn't nothing like that," he said. "I ended up getting a little bit of money. I was blessed to get what I got."

Was his stroke at a relatively young age related to the head banging he did in his football career? Or was it his predisposition to high blood pressure combined with not taking his meds? Carthon said he was never told by his doctors that football was the cause of his stroke, and he wasn't ready to say it himself.

Parcells consistently checks in with him. When Pepper Johnson was the linebackers coach on Mike Singletary's staff with the Memphis Express in the short-lived Alliance of American Football league in 2019, he moved in with Carthon in Jonesboro and made the one-hour drive each way twice a day. They had a lot to catch up on. The '86 Giants always enjoyed being around each other.

They also always found a little something to tease each other about.

"Maurice Carthon—he would love his clothes, and he protected them like they were gold," Simms said.

One day after practice, Carthon got all dressed up.

"Where are you going?" Simms asked.

"We're going to this club," Carthon said.

"Man, there's going to be music and dancing," Simms said.

"I'm going to dance, but I'm not going to move. You think I'm going to sweat in my suit?" Carthon said.

Recalling the conversation, Simms can't stop laughing.

"He didn't want to ruin that suit," Simms said.

In so many ways, they don't make them like Carthon anymore.

WILLIAM ROBERTS IS part of a group he calls "The Originators," the nearly two dozen Giants who played on the first two Super Bowl championship teams. That's opposed to "Eli's Group," the foundation of the Giants third and fourth championship teams more than twenty years later. Roberts was a versatile backup to the Suburbanites on the '86 team and a starter at guard on the '90 team.

Carson and Martin retired after the 1988 season. Morris went to play for Belichick in Cleveland in 1991. Marshall signed with the Jets in 1993. Banks signed with Washington in 1993. Taylor and Simms retired after the 1993 season. Jim Burt went to the 49ers in 1989. Bobby Johnson was traded to the Chargers in 1987. Bavaro signed with Belichick and the Browns in 1992.

Roberts was among the twenty-two players on the roster of the '86 and '90 teams. And by 1994, Roberts and Erik Howard were the last remaining players from the '86 team. It was the last year with Big Blue for each. Howard played two years for the Jets before Parcells got there. Roberts went to New England in 1995 to play two years for Parcells and then squeezed one last season out of his career with Parcells in his first year with the Jets in 1997.

"Bill told me, 'You're like a dog with a big bone. You won't let it go,'" Roberts said.

He helped spread the Parcells gospel in the locker room with the Patriots and Jets. He became part of his inner circle. He was a Parcells Guy. At the end of the '97 season, Parcells had the talk with Roberts. It was time to retire. "That's it, kid," Parcells said. "I'm going to let you go."

Following the victory in Super Bowl XXI, Roberts and Pepper Johnson went to the middle of the field at the Rose Bowl, placed their helmets on the grass, and did a silly dance called the dog, which they learned at a fraternity party when they were teammates at Ohio State. Roberts lives in Miami now and is an upbeat person, despite being on disability for football injuries he suffered to his knees, hips, and neck. He walks as much as he can to stay active. His unique gray beard is an instant conversation starter. He braids the hair around his chin, and it hangs all the way down to his chest.

Roberts had a health scare in 2002 that doctors told him was not related to football, but he's still not sure. He had a seizure and passed out. Didn't think much of it. Then it happened again. Then he thought a lot about it. He went for an MRI. The diagnosis: a blockage the size of a peach pit on the frontal lobe of his brain. Doctors told him that was the cause of the seizures. The frontal lobe controls memory, judgment, and motor tasks. Roberts had it removed and followed the surgery with chemotherapy and radiation "as a precaution," he said. "The tumor was benign."

"We just needed to extract as much as we could without having any damage," he said. "Since then, it's been okay."

The '86 Giants are fortunate: just one of their crew has passed away. Wide receiver Stacy Robinson, an enormously popular player who became an executive in the NFL Players Association, died of multiple myeloma, a blood cancer, at the age of fifty in 2012. Robinson won two rings with the Giants but didn't get to ring the bell in the hospital, the tradition for patients who are cancer-free. Ten teammates traveled to Maryland for his funeral. Three members of Parcells's staff have died: offensive coordinator Ron Erhardt, defensive line coach Lamar Leachman, and defensive backs coach Len Fontes.

Carson makes certain group photos are taken at the end of every reunion to preserve the moment. The reality is, nobody is sure who will be alive the next time they all get together. Just seeing one another makes them feel better, makes them feel younger. It takes them right back to 1986. "It's like medicine, treatment, therapy," Roberts said. "It's a strong dosage."

Burt had five surgeries on his back during his career and three more after he retired. On the thirty-year anniversary of the '86 championship, Burt and Oates each had stem cells injected into their knees. Burt also had stem cells injected into his shoulders. Oates has endured more than thirty surgeries, most of them after his career, including a knee replacement.

He became a lawyer and is the president of the NFL Alumni Association—an important position once held by Martin—and like many offensive linemen after they retire, he dropped a lot of weight. He played at 290 pounds and is down to 220. "I've had lots of surgeries, but all orthopedic stuff," Oates said. "My elbows, my knees, my back, yeah they suck, but you know, I have nothing to complain about."

Players see one another year-round at charity events, reunions, and autograph signings. Taylor, who is very much in demand, came up from Florida for a signing in New Jersey late in the fall of '22 and spent time at the event with Simms and Bavaro. It's a great opportunity to check up on one another and ask about who they've been in touch with recently. Word spreads fast if a member of the brotherhood is in trouble.

The '86 Giants are nearly unanimous: Offensive lineman Brad Benson is the teammate they are most worried about as the fortieth anniversary of the championship closes in. If there were an official count, Benson would lead the '86 Giants in post-football career maladies. "I call him Mr. Potato Head," Banks said. "Everything has been replaced." Benson made it through his ten-year career with the Giants without requiring one surgery or missing one practice due to injury. He's more than made up for it with a list of problems since he retired after the 1987 season that would crash the WebMD site.

Carson started a GoFundMe page in March 2022 designed to help Benson with his medical expenses. Benson had back surgery in 2012 that lasted fourteen hours. It was a front-to-back procedure—a laminectomy—in which he was cut open from the front. And the back. Surgeons trimmed the discs. The best he's been able to do after the surgery is walk with a noticeable limp. He's had his hips replaced. He needed a revision on one of them.

"Being a retired player is not for sissies," he said.

He recites his surgeries as if he's ordering off a menu. "Three hips . . . two backs . . . two necks . . . ," he said.

Benson has sought professional help for bouts of depression. When he was told that Bavaro had been diagnosed with atrial fibrillation and needed an ablation procedure to remove tissue, he said, "Yeah, I had that, too." He was diagnosed with lung cancer not long after his father died from the disease. Benson never smoked cigarettes and said his doctors in Boston called to tell him he had cancer and it was not caused by chewing tobacco when he played. The cancer showed on a myelogram test he was having done on his spine.

"You need to get to a hospital right now," his doctor said.

"Scared me to death," Benson said.

He was admitted to Memorial Sloan Kettering Hospital in Manhattan and was treated and released within forty-eight hours.

"Why me? What the fuck?" Benson asked one of his doctors when the surgeries began to pile up.

"What did you expect?" the doctor said.

"Not everybody has had this many surgeries," Benson said.

He remembers a concussion he suffered early in his career when he was on the punt coverage team and got hit from behind as he was running downfield. "My head hit the ground," he said. "I'm telling you, I had no idea where I was." Benson recalls a specific play against the Rams called "Flow 38," which linebacker Carl Ekern was able to diagnose. Benson, who was playing tackle at the time, said. "He hit me right on the chin. I guarantee you those neck surgeries are from that play." Ekern played thirteen years in the NFL and retired after the 1988 season. Two years later, he died from head injuries suffered in a car accident in California.

I met with Benson at his sprawling Rainbow Run farm in Hillsborough, New Jersey, in 2017, where he raises hay for horses. His teammates are hoping his financial problems won't cost him his property. He was an overachiever from Penn State who eventually found a home at left tackle, had brutal battles with Dexter Manley of Washington and Harvey Martin of the Cowboys, and helped keep his pal Simms on his feet. But he has paid the price with the deterioration of his body.

No doubt his physical issues resulted from his football career. "I was on the badminton team at Penn State for a while," he laughed. "You can blame it on that if you'd like."

Then, getting serious, he said, "I couldn't play badminton anyway. It would have interfered with the wrestling season." He did wrestle at Penn State.

Offensive linemen are anonymous until they get flagged for holding. They push ahead on running plays, backpedal on pass plays, and look like hell after games. Benson was the third-longest-tenured Giant by 1986. Only Martin and Carson had arrived before Benson in 1978, after he was originally drafted by the Patriots in the eighth round one year earlier.

Benson was distinguishable by the big, white bandage across the bridge of his nose on game days to cover and control the bleeding from a nasty cut that split open every week. He had plastic surgery during his career. The game day bandage made him look tough, and it once saved him a speeding ticket.

Benson and his wife Lisa were adopting a child from an agency in Cherry Hill in the southern portion of New Jersey less than two months before the Giants would play in Super Bowl XXI. The boy was born on December 8. Benson instructed the agency to call him on the Giants' main phone line when it was time for him and Lisa to pick up the baby and to ask for Eddie Wagner, the locker room manager, who would come get him. Benson was in an offensive line meeting with his coach Fred Hoaglin on December 11 when Wagner knocked on the door to inform Benson that the adoption agency was on the phone. It was time to take his son home. Before he left the stadium, he called Parcells to tell him he was leaving and why.

"Couldn't this wait until after practice?" Parcells said.

"Really?" Benson said. "If I tell these social workers that I can't come and pick this child up because I'm at work, they're going to boot my ass off the roster—their roster."

"Well, do what you have to do," Parcells said.

Benson owned a Jaguar dealership, but that week he was driving a Mercedes. He had won the use of the Mercedes for being player of the week after handling Manley in the biggest game of the season the previous Sunday in Washington, limiting him to three tackles and no sacks. As another souvenir from the game, the bridge of his nose was split wide open again. Benson had to drive 30 miles north to pick Lisa up at their home in Tuxedo, New York, and then 120 miles south to Cherry Hill, New Jersey, to pick up their baby boy, whom they named Tyler.

"He was our Super Bowl baby," Benson said.

His mind was racing. So was his car. He was pulled over by a Pennsylvania state trooper for speeding.

"What are you doing going 90 miles an hour?" the trooper said.

"We're adopting a child," Benson said, hoping for a little compassion.

"*I know you*," the cop said.

"Yeah," Benson said.

"You're the guy with the nose from the Giants!" he said.

Benson wanted to say, "We all have noses," but with the officer's ticket book in his hand and fearing his excessive speed could result in his car being towed, it was not the best time to be a smart-ass. He not only avoided a ticket, but the state trooper escorted him until he crossed state lines into New Jersey so he would not get stopped again. "What a great guy," Benson said.

He was the right tackle during the lowest moment in Giants history: the famous Pisarcik fumble. Instead of kneeling out the final seconds against the Eagles in 1978, offensive coordinator Bob Gibson ordered quarterback Joe Pisarcik to hand off to Larry Csonka. It was a bad exchange, and the ball hit the ground and bounced right up to Eagles cornerback Herm Edwards, who returned it twenty-six yards for the winning touchdown. Pisarcik went straight to Newark Airport after the game to catch a flight to Fort Lauderdale in an attempt to avoid the negativity. That turned out to be impossible. The next day, as Gibson was getting fired, Pisarcik was lying on the beach and looked up to see a man standing over him. He was a Giants fan who demanded an explanation why he didn't take a knee. "The Fumble" led to a complete revamping of the organization with the hiring of George Young and Perkins. It took eight more years, but Benson was finally playing in the Super Bowl. He had become an established left tackle and was rewarded with his first and only Pro Bowl.

The morning after the Super Bowl, the eight Giants in the Pro Bowl flew from Los Angeles to Honolulu. There was a gentleman's agreement among the linemen selected for the game to go light on the physical contact in practice and the game. No need to get injured in a meaningless exhibition. "Dennis Harrah, a guard from the Rams, and

Bob Golic, a defensive tackle with the Browns, were eating sushi and drinking beer together in the days before the game," Benson recalled. "One of them came off the ball harder in the game than the other one thought they should. The very first play, there's a fucking fistfight in the middle of the field."

Benson was a new daddy. He brought his wife and son to Honolulu, along with his sister-in-law to do the babysitting. He had his parents and in-laws in Pasadena for the Super Bowl. The Pro Bowl in the '80s was a bit more than the glorified practice the game later became before its demise, but Benson wasn't looking to pick up any new injuries after a Super Bowl season. Players rotate in and out of the Pro Bowl, but every time Benson looked up, Broncos defensive end Rulon Jones was staring across the line at him. Benson had just faced him seven days earlier in the Super Bowl and held him to four tackles and no sacks. If Jones considered the matchup the fifth quarter of Super Bowl XXI, Benson did not. "He was still pissed off," Benson said. "So, he was coming up the field pretty hard. I didn't need any of that."

Benson became more of a celebrity after his career than he was as a member of the Suburbanites. For a while, he owned a Hyundai dealership in South Brunswick, New Jersey, and he narrated commercials played during drive time on WFAN in New York, the most listened to all-sports station in the country. He wrote the commercials with a friend who lived in California, and they mixed in humor, politics, and R-rated material.

"It was my calling card," Benson said.

After Giants Stadium was knocked down following the 2009 season, Benson bought one set of the goalposts and displayed it on the grounds outside his Hyundai dealership. He invited listeners to visit his "forty-foot erection." It was cringeworthy to executives in the Giants organization who knew Benson and regretted he had stooped to that level to sell cars.

Benson sold Bill Belichick a used Mitsubishi when he was coaching for the Jets. Belichick kept it at his vacation home in Nantucket. He sold cars to McGriff and Carson. Benson eventually sold his automobile dealerships and no longer keeps a high profile. He had problems with his younger son Clint, who received three years' probation in 2016 for an alcohol-related hit-and-run automobile accident three years earlier; he hit a man walking away from his car after Clint Benson was confronted about reckless driving.

Brad Benson's teammates from the '86 Giants are pitching in to help get his finances in order, in addition to the fund Carson initiated. There's not much they can do about all the injuries that have worn down his body, but he has no regrets about playing.

"At the end of the day, I wouldn't trade it," he said.

Benson squeezed every last bit out of his body to last as long as he did in the NFL. The pressure to perform at a high level is immense, but it's not exclusive to the players.

5

FROM SEA GIRT WITH LOVE

Just across from the home team locker room under the lower-level stands of Giants Stadium was a row of reserved parking spots with enough room for five cars. The spots were so valued that not even Lawrence Taylor or Phil Simms could get one.

The east side tunnel facing Manhattan is where Wellington Mara, George Young, and Bill Parcells would drive in, take a quick right turn, slowly navigate sixty yards through the bowels of the stadium and turn left into their assigned spots surrounded by huge support beams. Parcells's car was always present when the players arrived in the morning and when they left at the end of the day. Young's car was big like him, and he was at the stadium every day unless he was attending an NFL meeting or had left at the end of the week to scout a college game. Mara was there most days after driving the sixty minutes across the bridge from his home in Rye in Westchester County, New York. He never moved to New Jersey after he relocated the team to the swamps of East Rutherford in 1976. His oldest son, John, who is now the Giants co-owner and team president, and his brothers Chris and Frank, who work for the team, have kept with family tradition and also remained in Westchester.

Parcells and his coaches worked into the evening hours four nights a week grading game footage, incessantly watching and rewinding film of the next opponent, and formulating the game plan to present to the players on Wednesday morning. Philadelphia's Dick Vermeil, down the Jersey Turnpike, camped out in his office at the rat-infested Veterans Stadium more often than he slept in his own bed at his home in Bryn Mawr, just an eighteen-mile trip. He thought the commute ate up too much valuable time away from preparation. Parcells didn't sleep in his office, but he still put in extremely long hours.

The difference in the appearance of an NFL coach from the beginning of training camp in July to the end of the season in December or January is striking. It's worse than dog years. By the completion of the seven-month grind, they've aged more than seven years. They are so obsessed with football and so insecure about their jobs, they rarely have an outlet to relieve stress. They are out of touch with what's going on in the world. They eat on the run and don't sleep enough. They are worn out, mentally drained, and badly in need of a beach vacation by Halloween.

Parcells didn't take great care of himself physically when he was coaching the Giants. He was too heavy and smoked too much. At least he had an escape to make sure he didn't mentally break down. Once or twice a season in the eight years he was head coach of the Giants, he would turn off the lights in his office on the street level of the stadium, walk down the one flight of stairs to his parking spot and get behind the wheel of his luxury Cadillac. It was 8:30 p.m. He would back up, make a left turn to the east side tunnel and maneuver through the stadium parking lot to the south entrance of the New Jersey Turnpike instead of heading home to Upper Saddle River on Route 17 North. He'd take the Turnpike to the Garden State Parkway south to Exit 98, and then it was just a couple of miles to Sea Girt on the Jersey Shore.

Giants Stadium to Sea Girt driving time: sixty-five miles, just over an hour.

Sea Girt was Parcells's happy place. Even at 10 p.m. Even for just seven precious hours.

Growing up, Parcells vacationed in Sea Girt with his family, and he bought a place there on Boston Boulevard a few houses from the Atlantic Ocean for $800,000 not long before he got back into coaching with Dallas in 2003, when Jerry Jones dangled a four-year, $17 million contract. They met at Teterboro Airport in New Jersey on Jones's private plane with the Cowboys blue star on the tail. The house went to his wife Judy following an amicable divorce settlement in 2002. The Cowboys money came after the split. Judy Parcells sold the house in 2019 for $1.8 million and purchased another in Sea Girt. One of Parcells's daughters lives in Sea Girt and another lives in the next town over in Manasquan. When Parcells makes his annual drive north from Tequesta to Saratoga, he stops off in Sea Girt to spend time with his family.

Bill and Judy were married forty years and have three daughters. Parcells admits he too often prioritized football over family. In the times he escaped his Giants Stadium office during the season and drove to the shore, he stayed the night. He didn't yet have a beach house, didn't stay in a hotel or with friends.

His visits to the beach town would be a fun premise for a reality show for NFL coaches. Parcells spent the night homeless. He never told anybody in the Giants organization—management, coaches, or players—about the excursions. When he reached Sea Girt, he sat on a bench on the boardwalk on the easternmost end of Beacon Street near a pavilion next to a pay phone. He gave the number to Judy in case she wanted to check up on him "so she doesn't think I'm fucking around," Parcells said.

He simply sat on the bench, soaking in the cool fall evening air, and didn't worry about the running game or the pass rush. He didn't think about NFC East coaches Tom Landry, Joe Gibbs, or Buddy Ryan. He looked out at the ocean, up at the moon, and Sunday's game for a brief period seemed as far away as the stars. When he got tired and could no longer keep his eyes open, he slept on the boardwalk bench or walked back to his car to get some rest. It's fortunate this was the pre–social media days or one of Parcells's overnight beach sleepovers would have been discovered, with his picture splattered all over Twitter. *TMZ* would have been tipped off that the coach of the freakin' New York Giants was sleeping on a bench at the beach and a reporter would have stuck a camera in his face, with a groggy Parcells telling them to "fuck off." His nickname was "Tuna," and it's not hard to imagine a New York tabloid headline in 72-point type: "AWOL Tuna Washed Up on Jersey Shore."

"I didn't walk the boardwalk. I would just be sitting on the bench relaxing," he said. "That was a peaceful place. You start to wind down a little. So, I'd sit there and might even lie on the bench and go to sleep. You know that [Southwest Airlines] commercial, 'You wanna get away?' I know exactly what they mean."

The Sea Girt police were familiar with Parcells and left him alone unless he was in the mood to chat. "I wasn't causing any trouble," he said. "This wasn't against the law." He was clearing his head, temporarily removing himself from the pressure of the season, and listening to the waves make sweet music smacking against the shore. It was heaven. He was not concerned for his safety fast asleep on a bench at 3 a.m. "Sea Girt is a very private small town," Parcells said. "There's not much activity at night. Especially during the school year it's a pretty quiet place."

At 5 a.m., before the sun would rise to warm up the Atlantic, Parcells would slip into a bathing suit and go for a dip in the ocean. Swimming at that early hour in the dark without a lifeguard is not recommended and potentially dangerous, but the cold salt water was invigorating. He would towel off, get dressed, stop for coffee, and be back in his office by 7 a.m. He didn't bother to shower in the coaches' locker room when he arrived at the stadium.

The ocean was his shower.

"If I would have known he was doing that shit, I would have had him put in a mental hospital," Lawrence Taylor said.

"Never heard that one. No," George Martin said.

Parcells would sleep in his office only after night games on the road, especially if the team plane landed at 5 a.m. after a West Coast game. He and the coaches would go straight from the airport to the stadium. He would work all morning, then instruct his assistant Kim Kolbe he was going to take a nap and to wake him after an hour. Home games were better. He would unwind at Manny's in Moonachie for dinner with his family, and it would be a happy crowd if the Giants won. "I don't drink, but after a game, I might have ten beers," he said. "I mean, not all the time, but you got to get away for a second, you know?"

Bill Belichick owns a vacation home in Nantucket, a small island thirty miles from Cape Cod and a hundred miles from Foxborough. Following mandatory minicamp in mid-June, coaches and players shut it down until training camp. Belichick often spends his down time in Nantucket on his boat "VIII Rings," but it doesn't provide the instant getaway Parcells had with Sea Girt. Travel time for Belichick from his office to Nantucket is three-and-one-half hours, including a ferry ride from the mainland to the island. Before the weather warms up in the offseason, Belichick often spends weekends at his townhouse in Jupiter, Florida. Boston provides plenty of things to do if Belichick needs a night out, and besides, he is not a likely candidate to sleep on the boardwalk anyway.

The '86 Giants had no way of knowing it, but Parcells and Belichick were the two best coaches ever to work together on any NFL staff, or at least since Vince Lombardi and Tom Landry were the coordinators for the Giants in the 1950s. Their personalities and skill sets could not be more different. Parcells was engaging, and Belichick didn't have the time, desire, or personality to show a lighter side. At least publicly. He loosens up when he's with friends. Parcells was very good with the Xs and Os, and was an elite game manager and motivator. Belichick was a savant with strategy, and as a head coach, he's also excellent at managing a game. Parcells was a big picture CEO. Belichick's strength even when working for Parcells was his attention to even the smallest detail.

Belichick was just twenty-nine years old when Parcells joined the Giants in 1981 as defensive coordinator. Belichick was working with the special teams. They had cubicles in the same office, and that's when they really got to know each other. Parcells was impressed with Belichick's knowledge about the defense and asked head coach Ray Perkins whether he could use him on Sundays to help with personnel groupings. Perkins agreed. Starting in 1983, when he succeeded Perkins, Parcells gave Belichick even more responsibility, eventually promoting him to defensive coordinator in '85.

Parcells was a people person. He instinctively knew how to piss off his players just enough, getting them fired up to play. He enjoyed kibitzing in the locker room in the morning and discussing life with the early arrivals. Parcells delegated responsibility to his assistants, but his fingerprints were still on everything. He was entertaining with the media, enjoyed sparring with the huge group of New York reporters covering the team, and he was informative at his press conferences, unlike Belichick, who has perfected the art of the nonanswer in New England.

The Giants offensive line in 1986 was composed of five white guys: Brad Benson, Billy Ard, Bart Oates, Chris Godfrey, and Karl Nelson. That inspired Parcells to come up with a nickname: the "Suburbanites." "It was not intended to be a compliment," Oates said.

If Parcells was insinuating they were soft, they countered by developing into a strong part of the team. The Suburbanites nickname caught on and became a big deal. Parcells came up with another nickname for his O-line that definitely was not flattering. The comeback from a 17–0 halftime deficit at Candlestick Park late in the 1986 season featured Bavaro's memorable play that inspired the Giants to an unlikely 21–17 victory. In that game, however, the Giants had no success running the ball. They totaled just 13 yards on the ground. Parcells's new nickname for the linemen?

"Club 13," Oates said.

When the Giants beat San Francisco by 46 points a few weeks later in the divisional round of the playoffs, the Giants ran for 216 yards. Mission accomplished.

"There were times I just couldn't stand Bill," Oates said.

Belichick was a grinder. He won over the Giants veterans with his preparation and in-game adjustments. As a Giants assistant, he didn't intimidate the players and the media like he's done for two decades in New England. Once he went to New England, he protected every last bit of information. If a player was on the injury report with an ankle sprain, he wouldn't say which ankle. His repetitive nonanswers, like "We did what we thought was best for the team" and "It is what it is" and "We're on to Cincinnati" became famous. Yet it was common in the Giants locker room after victories for Belichick to be asked by a reporter to draw up a defensive alignment that produced a turnover or big play. He would enthusiastically take the reporter's notebook and pen and diagram plays. He would rather give up one of his beloved hoodies than do it now, although he does take to his "Belestrator" to break down interesting plays of an opponent on his weekly television show in Boston.

The eight years Parcells was the Giants head coach, they were as well coached as any team in the Super Bowl era. It was not only Big Bill and Little Bill. The staff from 1983 to 1990 was packed with future NFL head coaches: Belichick, Tom Coughlin, Romeo Crennel, Al Groh, and Ray Handley, as well as a former head coach, Ron Erhardt. "You know, we weren't playing solitaire there," Parcells said. "I was lucky to have a pretty good staff."

The years have provided Parcells and Belichick perspective about what they've meant to each other. Parcells gave Belichick a running start by handing over a defense built around Taylor, which accelerated his growth as a coach. Parcells's expertise was on defense, and once he became comfortable that Belichick completely grasped the 3-4 scheme he installed in 1981, he gave him near-complete autonomy. Parcells worked hard to become a good offensive coach, just as Belichick did in New England, but he trusted Erhardt to run that side of the ball. That allowed Parcells to oversee the entire team.

The key to the Giants success was that Parcells and Belichick needed each other and relied on each other. The Giants were a dominant team in 1986 because they had a dominant defense.

"I tried to do my best every day to help the team in my role. My dad taught me that," Belichick said. "When I started coaching, I was the youngest coach in the NFL. Now, I'm one of the oldest. Both have their benefits, but it was certainly easier to relate to people your own age. On the other hand, I didn't have the experience that some other coaches had. I tried to learn quickly. Fortunately, I worked for a great defensive coach that knew fundamental football as well as any other coach. Bill deserves to be in the Hall of Fame for his leadership and ability to coach fundamental football. Nobody, and I mean nobody, was a better fundamental coach than Bill. In addition, Bill was great at figuring out how to win as a team each week. He simplified things and made everyone understand what it took to win each week—and he was always right. Whatever I lacked in experience, I was smart enough to watch and learn from Bill—how to handle a team and how to coach a defense to be fundamentally sound."

Two of Parcells's many oft-repeated catch phrases were "I go by what I see," and "You are what your record says you are." By those standards, Belichick's had the better career. Parcells was an NFL head coach for nineteen seasons but didn't win one playoff game in the seven years he coached without Belichick on his staff. Belichick won six Super Bowls without Parcells and also beat him in a playoff game when he was in Cleveland and Parcells was in New England. Belichick deserves the credit for drafting Tom Brady in the sixth round in 2000 and developing him into the greatest quarterback in NFL history. Parcells won Super Bowls with Phil Simms, the best quarterback in Giants history along with Eli Manning, and with Jeff Hostetler, who played the best football of his life down the stretch of the 1990 season, after Simms broke his foot.

Belichick's finest stretch for the Giants came in the 1990 playoffs when he dramatically changed his defense each week. He played a 4-3 against the run-heavy Bears, a 3-4 against Joe Montana's West Coast passing game, and, most famously, only two defensive linemen and nine defenders flooding the passing lanes to stop Jim Kelly's high-scoring no-huddle K-Gun offense in Super Bowl XXV against

Buffalo. The idea was to bait the Bills into running future Hall of Famer Thurman Thomas and give up yards on the ground rather than big chunks in the air. Prior to the game, Belichick told the defense if Thomas ran for 100 yards, the Giants would win. That went against the competitive instincts of his prideful defense, but Belichick wanted Kelly to throw the ball, force incompletions and quick possessions while intimidating and punishing Buffalo's receivers.

"The Buffalo Bills had that newfangled offense," Taylor said. "And Belichick comes in there talking, 'We're only going to rush two people. If we blitz, it's going to be three people.' I'm like, 'Get the fuck out of here.' But hey, it worked. He said we can't stop Thurman Thomas. Let him run. Let him do what he wants. From the 20 to the 20, let him run all he wants. Once you get to the red zone, then we are going to tighten down. He had 140-some yards rushing. The quarterback? Do what you do."

The Giants were not going to allow Kelly and wide receivers James Lofton and Andre Reed, all future Hall of Famers, to beat them to the trophy. "We didn't let that shit happen," Taylor said. Lofton had one catch for 61 yards, and Reed had eight catches for 62 yards, but the Giants put some vicious hits on Reed and pummeled him as he ran across the middle. Thomas ran fifteen times for 135 yards, and the Giants won 20–19 when Scott Norwood's 47-yard field goal sailed wide right with four seconds remaining. Kelly threw the ball thirty times, which was a lot in that era (and that was after scoring 51 points one week earlier in the AFC Championship Game against the Raiders). The Giants played ball control to keep the ball away from Kelly. The Bills countered with their hurry-up scheme but could not sustain drives—the Bills had just one possession over four minutes—and New York controlled the ball for a Super Bowl record 40:33. It was a brilliant defensive game plan by Belichick and overall strategy by Parcells.

The key was Taylor and Banks buying in. Belichick moved cornerback Everson Walls to safety and had him call the defensive signals, and he made a game-saving open-field tackle on Thomas on the Bills' final drive, preventing Norwood from having an easier field goal attempt. The three playoff games accentuated Belichick's creativity and the faith Parcells had in him. "Well, it's like having a top lieutenant," Parcells said. "First of all, it's the hardest job on the staff when the boss's area of expertise is what you are doing. After a year or so, I knew I didn't have to worry about it. Bill is very cerebral. He's got a lot of ideas and his mind races. Sometimes, I had to try to keep it a little simpler than maybe he wanted. But he had some good ideas that we used a lot. We both knew the subject matter. So, the conversations we had were very short and to the point."

As the defense evolved in 1986, Parcells gave Belichick the freedom to innovate. They spoke the same language. Parcells's staff was so good he didn't have to coach the coaches. Especially Belichick. "I was relying on him," he said. "I certainly understand that he was a very, very important and vital piece of the puzzle for me."

Parcells went on to coach the Patriots, Jets, and Cowboys and run football operations for the Dolphins. Now that he's retired, he bleeds Big Blue. Belichick's greatest years have been in New England, where he not only tripled the number of Super Bowls that Parcells won but will likely finish his coaching career with the most victories in NFL history and be remembered as the league's all-time best coach. When NFL Films followed Belichick around for the 2009 season for a two-part *A Football Life* documentary, it was the last year of Giants Stadium, the scene of so many great victories for the Parcells-Belichick Giants. The Patriots were playing the Giants in a preseason game on September 3 in the Meadowlands, and hours before the teams arrived, Belichick took the film crew on a nostalgic tour of the Giants locker room. The only time Belichick typically shows his emotional side is when he's yelling at officials during a game or hugging players after winning the Super Bowl. But in the interview with NFL Films, his voice cracked, and he was teary-eyed reminiscing about his twelve years with the Giants.

Belichick gave a rare peek behind his steel curtain. Even recalling that moment in the film more than ten years later revealed his sentimental side. "All the time I spent there, how much I grew and developed as a person and coach, how special the relationships were that I made—I get emotional just thinking about it now," he told me. "The Giants were terrible when I got there in 1979. I was so fortunate to be able to see how a championship team was built and rebuilt. When I left in 1991, I knew what greatness looked like, and I have tried to coach my teams to a comparable level ever since. I absolutely saw how it was done right, and I have been determined to follow that general blueprint for success."

After Parcells joined the Giants in 1981, he became a mentor to Belichick. Parcells was forty years old, nearly eleven years older than Belichick, and had a lot more experience. At that point in their lives, they were of different generations. They weren't best friends off the field but didn't need to be. Like any relationship, it had peaks and valleys, including a particularly famous and long-lasting falling out that began in January 2000.

At the time, Parcells was the head coach of the Jets, having left the Giants in 1991, then the Patriots in 1997, after a four-year run. The Jets were in the process of being sold by the estate of Leon Hess, who died in May 1999, to Woody Johnson for $635 million, and the imminent change in ownership scared both Parcells and Belichick. Belichick had been fired after five years in Cleveland and had two job offers: a reunion with Parcells or a spot on the staff of Jimmy Johnson, who had been hired to replace Don Shula with the Miami Dolphins. Belichick chose the familiarity of Parcells for what turned out to be Parcells's final season in New England. He then followed him to the Jets. Parcells informed Jets team president Steve Gutman immediately after the final game of the 1999 season against the Seahawks at Giants Stadium that he was stepping down as coach but would remain as general manager. The move automatically triggered a clause in Belichick's contract promoting him to head coach, with a three-year, $4.2 million contract. Hess also had paid Belichick a $1 million bonus a year earlier to turn down any head coaching opportunities.

Belichick, however, resented being manipulated by Parcells. Though he'd been hired in 1997 with the explicit understanding that he would eventually succeed Parcells as head coach, Belichick had expected to have a say in when the transition happened. With the team being sold, and his new position compromised by both an unknown new owner and his old boss remaining as GM, Belichick wanted to leave to coach the Patriots, who had fired Pete Carroll. After eight years with the Giants, one with the Patriots, and three with the Jets, Belichick wanted to get away from operating in Parcells's shadow, even though Parcells had pledged he would stay in the background in only a supporting role. By then, it was widely known that Patriots owner Robert Kraft wanted to bring Belichick back to New England. Parcells held a press conference the day after he informed Gutman he was stepping down. He said he would never coach again and that the media could write that on their chalkboards. The media was anticipating Belichick would follow Parcells to the podium. When that failed to materialize, Belichick sent word through the public relations staff that the day belonged to Parcells and he would speak Tuesday.

Three years earlier, Belichick had run interference for Parcells, moving with him from the Patriots to the Jets and agreeing to stand in as interim coach until a compensation deal was worked out between Hess and Kraft. It took six days. Belichick agreed to move to the Jets with Parcells only after Kraft denied him the opportunity to succeed Parcells as the Pats head coach, a job Belichick very much wanted. Kraft was fond of Belichick and in his heart wanted to hire him. Belichick had spent the 1996 season with Parcells in New England—the Pats lost to the Packers in the Super Bowl—and cozied up to Kraft. He explained behind-the-scenes football decisions, which Parcells had refused to do, and kept Kraft in the loop on things he was interested in. When Parcells and Kraft split, Kraft and his wife Myra took Belichick and his wife Debby out to dinner in Boston. Kraft explained why he couldn't promote Belichick. He had such a residual bitter taste from three years with Parcells (Kraft bought the Patriots following Parcells's first season in New England) that he needed a clean break from his coaching tree. He hired Carroll instead.

Belichick believed Parcells resigned so quickly after the final game to prevent him from leaving for New England. The Patriots sent a letter to the Jets first thing Monday morning requesting permission to interview him, which the Jets denied. Belichick resented the man who was supposed to be his mentor interfering in his career. Belichick's celebratory press conference to introduce him as the Jets coach was scheduled for 2:30 p.m. in the team meeting room on the second floor of Weeb Ewbank Hall at the Jets training facility. Belichick held a staff meeting that morning, but the sense in the building was something weird was about to happen. As Belichick later walked from his office to the press conference, he told his assistant coaches he was quitting, handed Gutman his resignation letter and rambled at his press conference for twenty-five minutes before taking questions.

On a plain piece of loose-leaf paper, Belichick scribbled a resignation letter and handed it to Parcells and Gutman before addressing the media. He read the letter in the press conference:

Due to various uncertainties surrounding my position as it relates to the team's new ownership, I've decided to resign as head coach of the New York Jets. I've given this decision very careful consideration. I would like to wish the entire New York Jets organization, the players, the coaching staff and the new ownership the very best of luck for a prosperous future.

He had written the resignation letter so quickly that he scribbled "HC of the NYJ," instead of spelling it out. Gutman was fuming as Belichick spoke. As Belichick walked out the side door and back to his office, Gutman stepped up to the podium and all but said Belichick was having a nervous breakdown. "We should have feelings of sorrow and regret for him and his family. He obviously has some inner turmoil," he said.

It became nasty and went to court, with the Jets winning. Parcells, in his capacity as Jets GM, eventually made a deal with Kraft to trade

Belichick to New England for a first-round draft pick just as Kraft was ready to give up his month-long chase and hire former Carolina Panthers coach Dom Capers. Belichick learned from Parcells about the fine art of manipulation.

"Shit happens in this business," Parcells said. "And a few things he did I didn't like. But he's had some guys do the same thing to him now, so he gets it." Carl Banks finished up his career playing the 1994 and 1995 seasons for Belichick in Cleveland. He went against the Patriots and Parcells three times, including a Belichick victory over Parcells in a wild-card playoff game following the '94 season. Before one of the games, Kraft walked over to Banks during warm-ups and quizzed him for twenty minutes about his experience playing for Belichick in New York and Cleveland. Banks gave him rave reviews, and Kraft followed up the next time the teams played. Kraft later told Banks their talks were instrumental in his decision to hire Belichick as head coach.

Parcells was generous providing Belichick with insight and advice on being a head coach in the years before he was hired by the Browns in 1991 and now serves as a sounding board with Belichick navigating the post-Brady era in New England. Parcells's message: every day new and impossible to anticipate problems show up on a head coach's desk, and you better be prepared to react quickly. "Bill was a great resource through the years on many different levels," Belichick said. "We worked well together and won a lot of football games." In the spring of 2022, Belichick sent Parcells a note that touched him. "It was just so nice and gracious," Parcells said. "It was very meaningful. We're both grateful. You know, I'm glad that I met him. My professional career wouldn't have been the same without him. That's how I feel."

Why does he think Belichick sent this note now after so many years? "Maybe he thinks I'm going to die soon," Parcells said. "You never know. I'm eighty-one years old and one of these days it's going to happen."

Parcells first met Belichick through his father, Steve Belichick, an assistant on the Naval Academy staff when Parcells was on the coaching staff at Army. They were in charge of exchanging game film and would see each other every week. Bill Belichick was still in college playing football and lacrosse at Wesleyan University and was just twenty-two years old when he met Parcells, who by then had moved on to defensive coordinator at Vanderbilt. Steve brought his son down after a game so he could introduce them.

"Bill and I formed a close friendship and professional relationship at the Giants over a number of years that grew over time," Belichick said. "Our professional relationship was always simple. He was the boss. If he wanted something done a certain way, I did it whether I agreed with it or not. He would listen to my opinion, but in the end, he had final say and I totally respected that. He made the decisions that were best for the team, and I had 100 percent confidence in Bill."

After Parcells was nearly fired after the 1983 season, Belichick accepted a position as the defensive backs coach on the Vikings staff of head coach Les Steckel, who had just been promoted from receivers coach after Bud Grant retired. It was a lateral move, but he received Parcells's blessing to take the job. Parcells was on shaky ground in New York and did not want Belichick to be swept out in a massive housecleaning if the Giants didn't win in 1984. Belichick visited the Vikings offices and decided it was a good fit. But just as career waffling by Parcells became his trademark, Belichick changed his mind and remained with Parcells. "After giving it serious thought, I wanted to be with Bill and do all I could to help the Giants win," Belichick said.

It was a wise career move. Steckel's military background didn't translate well to running a football team. He was disciplined and rigid and alienated his players. He had a 3–13 record and was fired after one season. Parcells turned things around in New York in 1984. The Giants were 9–7 and won a playoff game, and Parcells elevated Belichick to defensive coordinator after the season.

Belichick had proven himself to Parcells, which led to him proving himself to the players. Parcells destroyed any doubts GM George Young had about his ability to lead the Giants by bouncing back from his rookie season as a head coach and showing the job was not too big for him. Parcells and Young spent their last seven seasons together barely tolerating each other. But on the field, things got better and stayed that way. The more responsibility Parcells gave Belichick setting up the defensive game plan, the more the players believed in him. They were confident he was going to put them in the best position to succeed. The more he helped them succeed, the more money they made. That resulted in respect.

It's not as if Parcells and Belichick played good cop/bad cop with the players. They were both demanding. Belichick had a perpetual sour look on his face and was always convinced the next trainwreck was coming full speed down the tracks. That amused more than intimidated the defensive players. "There's a reason why Belichick's nickname was Doom," Taylor said, laughing.

He was a master at calling an audible from his game plan and didn't need to wait until halftime to do it. He would squat in front of the players on the bench, turn his whiteboard toward them and draw schemes upside down that produced immediate results. Taylor often improvised and was successful even if he disregarded his assignment, and Parcells and Belichick were flexible enough at L.T.'s urging to incorporate his ideas into the defense. The '86 Giants defense might not have reached the level of the 1985 Bears, but it was pretty close. And it had Taylor, better than any player on Chicago's formidable unit.

Belichick has climbed to unimaginable heights in his more than twenty years in New England. Walking away from the Jets, a team perpetually trying to find its way, was a brilliant career move. But his coaching roots are in New York. He created a dynasty in New England but agreed that the bond of the '86 Giants stands out. "The team was special—it had a special chemistry," he said. "There was a genuine love for each other and appreciation for what everyone was contributing. Taylor and Simms had great years—that had a lot to do with it. When they were going great, they tend to bring a lot of people with them. I don't mean to single them out, but they were special. We had a host of others, too. Parcells, Simms, and Taylor were unbelievable leaders and drove the team in a unique way. Hard to explain, but very, very special."

Parcells was unpredictable with his career decisions. The more Parcells won, the more he wavered on how much he had left in the tank. That agitated Belichick. He should have left a gas can in his boss's locker. Right after the Super Bowl XXI victory over Denver, Parcells attempted to jump to the Atlanta Falcons as coach/general manager. His power play took away from the joy of the moment for Wellington Mara and his family. Mara's friend, commissioner Pete Rozelle, stepped in at the Giants' insistence and enforced Parcells's contract. In the days leading up to the Giants Super Bowl victory over Buffalo following the 1990 season, the Giants knew they would be losing Belichick to the Cleveland Browns. He had interviewed with Browns GM Ernie Accorsi after the 1988 season at the Senior Bowl, and Accorsi was impressed enough to keep talking with Belichick and skip practice. But Cleveland decided to go with longtime NFL assistant Bud Carson, believing the team was Super Bowl ready and needed a veteran voice. Carson lasted just two seasons. Accorsi then recommended Browns owner Art Modell hire Belichick in 1991. Harry Carson, who was with Belichick for ten years in New York, wrote a letter of recommendation to Modell.

The Browns advanced to the AFC Championship Game in 1986 and 1987 and in Bud Carson's first season in 1989 but lost all three times to John Elway and the Broncos. The Browns fell apart in 1990, and Carson was fired after a 3–13 season. Belichick started off 6–10 in Cleveland then had back-to-back 7–9 seasons. He did not have many supporters in the Cleveland media. Belichick's press conferences were painful to watch. His dedication to secrecy was absurd, and he was clearly uncomfortable in front of large media groups. During his third season, Belichick demoted and then cut wildly popular hometown quarterback Bernie Kosar, a Browns icon, and went with Kosar's former University of Miami backup Vinny Testaverde, who developed into the first overall pick by the Bucs in the 1987 draft. The Browns made the playoffs in Belichick's fourth season in 1994 after an 11–5 year and beat the Patriots and Parcells in the wild-card game in Cleveland, but they lost in the next round in Pittsburgh.

Big things were expected of the Browns in 1995. They got off to a slow 4–4 start before a tsunami arrived. Modell sabotaged the season at the halfway point when he announced he was moving the team to Baltimore in 1996. He'd fought for years with the City of Cleveland, trying to secure public funding for a new stadium to replace rundown Cleveland Stadium. Modell complained he could not even get the leaky toilets fixed. He bought the Browns for just $4 million in 1961, helped negotiate the NFL's network television contracts that put millions in every owner's bank accounts, but cried poverty on the way out the door after he watched the city provide funds to help build a new baseball stadium and basketball arena.

In the Browns' final appearance in Cleveland in the next-to-last game of their fiftieth season, the officials twice in the fourth quarter flipped the offenses around from driving toward the Dawg Pound in the east end zone for fear of flying objects. "Security said it was getting too dangerous, but I really didn't notice anything except for a few explosions," Testaverde said in the locker room after the game.

The residents of the fabled Dawg Pound did rip out the bench seating and hurled the boards onto the field, along with golf balls and other assorted accessories. The Browns said goodbye with a victory over the Bengals, their only win in the eight games following Modell's announcement. Belichick was the first casualty. He was fired. Modell said he didn't want any of the negativity Belichick could never shake after cutting Kosar to follow him to Baltimore. Modell desired a clean slate and feared Belichick's presence could adversely impact the anticipated increased revenue and new stadium Baltimore was building for him. No coach, not Paul Brown, George Halas, or Don Shula, could have succeeded in Cleveland in 1995.

After eight years of working for Parcells and then becoming a head coach for five seasons, Belichick took a step back in his career and worked for Parcells again. But he did help repair the damage done to his reputation in Cleveland. Jim Burt, who was with Belichick for eight seasons with the Giants, believes "going back and being an assistant under Parcells, where you don't even have to piss him off and he's going to say something bad to you if he's in a bad mood" was difficult for Belichick after being his own boss for five years.

Parcells's own future with the Giants was a hot-button topic during his press conferences during Super Bowl week in January 1991 in Tampa. New York had just upset the 49ers in San Francisco 15–13 in the NFC Championship Game, eliminating the two-time defending champs on five field goals. Once again, they knocked Joe Montana out of the game, just as they had in the 1986 playoffs. Instead of Burt giving Montana a concussion, this time Leonard Marshall sent him out of the game in the fourth quarter after a vicious blindside hit that resulted in Joe Cool suffering a concussion, bruised sternum, bruised stomach, broken hand, and cracked ribs. The feeling outside the Giants organization was that if Parcells resigned immediately after the Super Bowl, then Belichick would be promoted, preempting his move to Cleveland. Presumably, Belichick had a vested interest in Parcells's decision. Belichick deserved to be the next man up if Parcells departed. Those inside the Giants organization knew Young didn't believe Belichick's personality translated well into being a good head coach. There was no immediate decision by Parcells after the Super Bowl. The Browns announced Belichick's hiring ten days later.

Once the head coach hiring season ended and the Browns introduced Belichick, it was assumed Parcells would return for his ninth season. He may not have liked Young, but he cared enough about Mara not to be vindictive and quit deep into the offseason. Three-and-one-half months after the Super Bowl, word started to leak late on the night of May 14 that Parcells was indeed stepping down. A press conference was called for the next day in the press lounge upstairs at Giants Stadium. Parcells was vague when pressed by the media for an explanation and denied it was health related. It wasn't until months later that he revealed issues with his heart led to his resignation. He ultimately had multiple surgeries. "I knew something

was wrong, but I wasn't sure what it was," Parcells said. "I was having more and more serious episodes. We didn't figure out until December what was going on." Parcells insists he was not being vindictive
and delaying his announcement because of his dislike for Young. "I
wouldn't have waited until May if I knew I was going to leave," he said.

The Giants were in a bind. It was two months before training
camp, and Parcells was gone, Belichick was gone, and wide receivers
coach Tom Coughlin had accepted a job as the Boston College head
coach in late December, stayed on for the playoffs, and was gone after
the Super Bowl.

Giants fans were rightfully livid. How could they lose Parcells
and Belichick in the same offseason? Now, two months before training
camp following their second Super Bowl season, they had neither to
help defend the title.

If Parcells was going to leave, why didn't he step away in time
for Young to replace him with Belichick? The answer: It didn't matter.
Young disliked Belichick even more than he disliked Parcells. Young's
ready list to replace Parcells had only one name: little-known running
backs coach Ray Handley, a math whiz who assisted Parcells on the
sidelines with clock management. Handley had the appearance and
demeanor of a high school history teacher. That's what attracted him
to Young, a former high school history teacher himself. Even if Belichick had remained with the Giants, Young likely would have coached
the team himself before promoting him. He thought Belichick was a
bad communicator and would not be able to command the attention of
an entire roster. Belichick didn't like Young, either. "I respected George
Young's position," Belichick said. "I didn't respect the way he handled
Bill after the 1983 season."

Late in the 1990 season, with all indications Parcells was going to
lose Belichick and Coughlin, he went to Young. "I specifically asked
him the question: You want me to keep these guys here? The answer
was no. Either one of them. That's the truth," Parcells said. "There
were two people George didn't like in terms of being a potential head
coach."

That was Belichick and Coughlin. Young was enamored with Handley, who turned out to be way over his head and mishandled the difficult Phil Simms versus Jeff Hostetler controversy between the Super Bowl–winning quarterbacks in 1991 and faced a defensive insurrection in 1992. He was fired after two seasons and replaced by Dan Reeves, who had lost to the Giants in Super Bowl XXI. Young's first choice to replace Handley was actually Coughlin, but he turned down the job, not wanting to leave Boston College after just two years. He would leave BC one year later to run the expansion Jacksonville Jaguars one year in advance of their first game. Long after Young had left the Giants and subsequently passed away a few years later, Coughlin coached the Giants from 2004 to 2015 and won two Super Bowls. Young's second choice in 1993 was Cowboys defensive coordinator Dave Wannstedt, who was talked out of the job by his best friend Jimmy Johnson, the Cowboys coach. Johnson didn't think it would be good for their friendship if they competed in the same division. Wannstedt was hired by the Bears. There was no chance Young would rehire Parcells, who got back into coaching in 1993 in New England after his medical issues had been addressed. Wellington Mara knew Reeves through Landry, a very close friend, and had interviewed him for the head coaching job before he hired Young, who hired Perkins. After Young couldn't lure Coughlin or Wannstedt to New York in 1993, Mara forced his hand and made him hire Reeves. Young was wary of Reeves's ability to work in the Giants structure with the general manager having final say. Reeves had run his own show in Denver for twelve years.

Young turned out to be right. Reeves was mostly miserable in his four seasons with the Giants, with only his first one a playoff year. The Giants were again looking for a head coach in 1997. Young might have been the only member of the Giants organization not upset when Parcells left six years earlier. And then he blocked Parcells 2.0 in 1997 when he was available after his falling out with Kraft in New England.

Parcells ended up with the Jets, but prior to the deal being finalized, there was a bizarre twist to the story.

"Wellington called me up," Parcells said. "He talked to me about the Giants a little bit."

Mara asked Parcells if he wanted to come back and coach the team he loved and led to two Super Bowl titles.

Initially, co-owner Robert Tisch didn't want Parcells. He didn't know him. He had purchased 50 percent of the team from Wellington's nephew Tim Mara, and Parcells was gone three months later. But knowing that Mara really wanted to bring him back, Tisch gave in and endorsed Parcells. Young, however, wanted no part of a Parcells sequel. His plan was to hire former Giants assistant Jim Fassel. When Young heard Mara and Tisch agreed on Parcells, he rushed down the hall to his office and called Fassel in his New Jersey hotel room where he had been waiting after he interviewed and quickly offered him the job. Mara was not aware of Young's call to Fassel when he marched into Young's office and asked him to offer the job to Parcells. Young informed Mara he had already extended the offer to Fassel. Mara was a man of integrity and didn't insist Young rescind the offer. Young also prided himself on his integrity but had just pulled a fast one on his bosses.

Would Parcells have gone back to work for Young rather than go to the Jets to coach the team and be his own boss? "I can't say that. It never got that far. I knew it wasn't going to happen with the Giants," Parcells said. "But here's what I can tell you. I always had a wonderful relationship with Wellington Mara until the day he died. I talked to him. I wrote him a letter when he was in the hospital. I have a high regard for him."

Parcells's closest contact with the Giants now is Ronnie Barnes, the head athletic trainer. He tries to get to a Giants game every couple of years during the fall when he's in Saratoga. He takes his former girlfriend's son, supplies him with Eli Manning gear he gets from the Giants, and drives three hours to MetLife Stadium. The boy is being raised by a single mother, and Parcells doesn't want him to miss out on the experience.

Belichick still has a soft spot for the Giants, and one of his close friends said if the timing and circumstances were right in the mid- to late 2010s, it was the only job in the NFL that could entice him to leave New England. He dismissed any thought of a return to New York because he believed the Giants front office and scouting department needed an overhaul and he didn't have the desire to go through a complete rebuild in his late sixties. "My goal has always been to help coach my team to a championship, not to leave and go somewhere else," Belichick said. "When Bill was the coach of the Giants, I had an opportunity to be a head coach in Cleveland. I was not looking to leave, but professionally, it was a great opportunity. My transitions in coaching were about timing and opportunity."

━━

ATTENTION TO DETAIL is what made Parcells and Belichick elite coaches. Whether it was Parcells having his punter run out of the back of the end zone for a safety late in the game rather than attempt a risky kick that could be blocked and recovered for a touchdown or Belichick sitting on the Giants team bus to Philadelphia devouring newspaper clips to find one bit of minutia he could use to his advantage, there was never a situation that caught the Giants coaches by surprise in 1986.

"I thank Parcells all the time," McConkey said. "I thought I knew what it was to be a champion. I didn't. I thought I was giving everything I had. I wasn't. He got more out of me than I ever thought possible."

McConkey's masterful job catching punts in the 25-mile-per-hour gusts of wind in the NFC Championship Game victory over Washington saved the Giants 100 yards of field position. Parcells referred to it as hidden yardage because it doesn't show up on the stat sheet. McConkey was just as crucial in the victory as Sean Landeta punting through the stiff wind. McConkey wasn't the best punt returner, but he would always catch the ball.

"This is going to sound a little egotistical and big headed and crazy, but I can honestly say at one point in my life, I could do something better than anybody on the face of the planet. Catch punts," he said. "Because if you're the best guy to catch punts in the NFL, you're probably the best in the world. And I think I was the best guy."

Parcells trusted McConkey, but if he thought his performance in the championship game was going to get him the benefit of the doubt in training camp seven months later, he quickly found out that was not in the coach's playbook. Parcells was demanding. Receivers coach Pat Hodgson called Parcells "a bear on the sidelines," during games. He was just as bad at practice. On the morning of the second day of two-a-days in the summer of 1987, McConkey caught a finger in the eye from a defensive back. He still had his shoulder pads on when he got in the car with Barnes and went to see an ophthalmologist in White Plains. He took his pads off in the car, and when they arrived at the doctor's office, he still could not open his eye. He was diagnosed with a scratched cornea and given antibiotic drops to take three times a day and a black patch to wear over his damaged eye.

The first thought leaving the doctor's office: he missed lunch, he was hungry, he was sweaty, but he better not miss practice. "It's no excuse," McConkey said. "One eye, black patch, no excuse." He stopped with Barnes at a 7-Eleven to pick up a sandwich, ate in the car, ran into the locker room, and put his pads and jersey back on for the afternoon practice. He was on the field just before Parcells blew the whistle to get started.

"Parcells is staring at me," he said. "He knew what was going on, but it was like, 'You're almost late.' Any other team, any other coach, you're off until your vision comes back, right? You at least have the afternoon practice off. It's Ronnie and me. We knew we had just won the Super Bowl, I'm better at catching punts than anybody on the planet, but we knew I had to get to practice."

McConkey surprisingly had little trouble catching passes from Simms and Hostetler that afternoon. As usual, he stayed afterward to field punts for as long as the punters wanted to kick the ball to him. Parcells watched intently. McConkey noticed his teammates parading from the locker room to the cafeteria for dinner. He was hungry, having missed a real lunch, and tired without a between-practices nap, and was still wearing his smelly gear from the morning practice. Once the punters were done, one of the ball boys who McConkey tipped all summer to fire up the JUGS machine after practice stayed late to send 60-yard missiles for him to field.

"I'm catching all these balls, and with one or two left, I dropped it, I tried to double catch it and it hits the ground," he said.

He was doing this all with one eye.

"Parcells screams at me as if I just fumbled away the Super Bowl," he said. "I'm thinking, 'You fucking big ass, I've been out here since eight in the morning.' I hated him. But the son of a bitch got me to focus so far beyond anything I was ever capable. That's what coaches do. What teachers do."

Belichick learned from Parcells that the smallest bit of intel can produce a victory, even a Super Bowl victory, and he took that with him to Cleveland and New England. When it's cold and rainy in Foxborough and the forecast for Sunday calls for a nasty New England winter day, Belichick takes his team to the outdoor practice fields with the Patriots indoor facility a few hundred yards away. If you have to play in it, you practice in it.

BY THE TIME the '86 Giants won the Super Bowl, they were convinced Belichick was going to be a very good head coach once he left the Parcells nest. Did they think he was going to win six Super Bowls and challenge Don Shula for the most victories in NFL history? Did the players know in real time as they began the 1986 season that they were being coached by two future Hall of Famers?

Hell, no.

Parcells, maybe. Belichick, come on.

Defensive tackle Curtis McGriff, who signed with the Giants as a rookie free agent in 1980, said when he arrived that Belichick was the Rodney Dangerfield of the Giants. He worked with special teams, had a short résumé, was only twenty-eight years old, younger than some of the players, and unknown to many of them. "He didn't bring a lot of clout to the table," McGriff said.

Taylor then and now believes Parcells is the best coach he's ever had. He came to like and greatly respect Belichick. He just never envisioned him as the best coach ever. "Who would have thought that little Doom would amount to anything like that?" Taylor said. "When he became defensive coordinator, I had a problem with that. Man, Belichick don't even know our names. What the hell? It was, 'Hey you, come here.' He can't be running the defense. But Bill Parcells had a lot of respect for him. He told me he does design the defenses and stuff like that. I thought that was interesting. And he has proven to be a great coach. I can't say nothing but give him praise."

Is he surprised Belichick has smashed so many coaching records? "You are in a way because of so many personalities he has to deal with, and Bill doesn't do personality very well," L.T. said. "But you're not surprised by the football knowledge this guy has. We can fuss and we can cuss during the week, but on Sunday everybody is standing around him because we know he has a plan." Martin was certain of one thing about Belichick's coaching future during his formative years with the Giants. "Well, we knew he wasn't going to be a public address announcer," he said. "Belichick has always been a man of few words."

He did know Belichick was focused on football and not much else. "He had initially stated that during the season, nothing comes between his obligations as a coach, not family, not anything, that is what he does," Martin said. "And when he said that, Harry and I looked at each other and said, 'Damn.' He was just one dimensional. He was totally focused on football. Period. He was in such a football zone that he separated himself from the crowd because of his burgeoning genius. Inevitably, he became what he is today. Does that surprise anyone? No. It seemed like it was almost predestined because that was the kind of dedication he had."

Carson helped organize the twenty-fifth anniversary reunion of the '86 team on June 11, 2011. They had a dinner at the Legacy Club, which serves as a Giants Hall of Fame, at MetLife Stadium. Fifty-one of the fifty-three players and seven coaches attended. Carson set the date for six weeks before training camps opened, enabling Belichick and others still coaching to make the trip. "When I started planning, I called Parcells. Then I called Belichick. And then I called Simms and then I called Taylor," Carson said.

They all said yes.

"Once I got those four, I refused to take no for an answer from anybody else," Carson said.

Hostetler was in Africa. Carson said he was on a church mission. Running back George Adams was the other player missing. He was taking his son Jamal—who later became a Pro Bowl safety—on college visits. The gathering was loud and jubilant, with jokes being told and stories embellished. "You fall right back into the locker room. That same dynamic existed thirty-five years ago, you go right back there," Oates said. "Everybody resumed the role that they had. Some may try to get out of their lane and you slap them right back."

The players and coaches were gathered eagerly waiting for one more person to walk into the room.

Footsteps were heard.

The mood changed.

The room got quiet.

"They did it out of tremendous respect," Simms said. "They couldn't wait to see him."

In walked Parcells.

He could still command a room. By then, Parcells was retired, and Belichick had won his first three Super Bowls in New England. "I feel really honored and special to know I was coached by two of the very best and that Belichick, at some point, might be recognized as the best head coach in football history," Carson said. "I think Belichick learned a lot from Parcells. And keep in mind, Belichick never really played. He got it rough from the guys he coached. You know, he's a guy who just played lacrosse."

He became a football genius, proving again the best football coaches are not often the best football players. "Back then, he looked like a California surfer dude. His hair was kind of long, he had the cut-off sleeves and was running around without any socks. It looked like he was ready to go to the beach," Leonard Marshall said. "But I knew he was destined for greatness."

He laughs at Belichick's appearance now. "He looks like a grumpy old man," he said.

Belichick is now considered more accomplished than Parcells. But on the '86 Giants, the hierarchy was well defined, and in Taylor's mind, it still is. "I know Belichick is racking up all kinds of accolades and championships, but he's still my number-two coach when it comes to Bill Parcells," he said. "Now number two ain't bad, but he's still my number two."

Burt was a serious football player on the field and a character off it. He might have been the last player on the defense who figured to bond with Belichick, but he felt a genuine chemistry with him. "Loved him. I love Belichick," Burt said. Belichick considered him an overachiever, which is how Burt viewed himself. "He was very appreciative when you played your ass off," Burt said. "So was Parcells, but Belichick was as hardcore as you could possibly get. More than Parcells. When I say hardcore. I never thought he could be a head coach. Ever. Parcells would get on guys to motivate them and then behind the scenes, he would put his arm around you. Belichick would never do that to anybody. He was like a stern military guy. But, hey, if you were one of his guys and you produced. . . . I loved the guy. I really did."

The Giants had a luncheon at Gallagher's restaurant in midtown Manhattan in 2006 to celebrate Carson's upcoming induction into the Hall of Fame. Parcells, Belichick, and Burt were there. Parcells cut Burt and tried to push him into retirement on the eve of training camp in 1988, expressing concern for Burt's back issues. Burt was insulted. He felt he had more football in him, signed with the 49ers, and won another Super Bowl. Before a highly anticipated game in 1990 against the Giants, Burt was still bitter and threatened to bowl over Parcells if New York ran a sweep near the Giants sideline. As Burt stood with his two former coaches at the luncheon, Belichick said to Parcells, "You got rid of Burt way too early." Burt has always appreciated Belichick having his back.

Even if Burt could deal with Belichick's quirky personality, he still didn't think it translated well to being a head coach. "You have to get guys to play for you. You have to get guys to buy into what you're doing, and Parcells was a master at it," he said. "So that's what I'm used to. Belichick wasn't into any of that. Belichick was all about can you play or can't play, this is how we're doing it and that was it. You can do that with most of the white guys. But some of the Black guys you can't do that with. There's a lot that goes into it. They didn't grow up with fathers and you have to massage those guys. Belichick is not a massage guy. I never thought he'd be able to handle it, and he handled it."

Players who left the Giants and went to play for other teams compared the coaching they were getting to what they had in New York. "Once you play for a coach who is that detail oriented, then you have a measuring stick of how to judge and rank other coaches," cornerback Mark Collins said.

He played his first five years for Parcells and Belichick, then two years for Handley, one year for Reeves, then three years for Marty Schottenheimer in Kansas City, before finishing up with one year with Mike Holmgren in Green Bay and one year with Dennis Erickson in Seattle. Collins was impressed playing for Reeves and Holmgren. "Then you get a guy like Marty Schottenheimer, who doesn't have a fucking clue," Collins said. After the Chiefs won the AFC West in 1995 and had a bye before the divisional round, Schottenheimer called Collins into his office. Schottenheimer had a reputation for running difficult practices, the primary reason Joe Montana lasted only two seasons in Kansas City after he was traded to the Chiefs in 1993. Collins tried to warn Schottenheimer about wearing out his players and to take care of their bodies at playoff time like Parcells did. "We've already got the division won," Collins said. "We're not killing each other for two and one half, three hours in practice. Right, Marty?"

But Schottenheimer knew only one speed. Kansas City, which finished as the No. 1 seed with a 13–3 record, then lost at home to the

Colts, who snuck into the playoffs at 9–7. Schottenheimer is the best regular season coach who never made it to the Super Bowl. His teams annually fell apart in January.

As Belichick gained his footing with the Giants, he had creative differences with Parcells. It would occasionally show up on NFL Films sideline footage with Parcells yelling at Belichick about a defense he wanted called and Belichick letting him know things were under control. It was not Mike Ditka versus Buddy Ryan on the staff of the wild '85 Bears. Those two hated each other. Ryan considered himself the co–head coach and wouldn't let Ditka near his defense. When Ditka was hired by George Halas in 1982, he forced him to keep Ryan, who created an offense versus defense divide in the Bears locker room.

Parcells was happy to give Belichick the responsibility to run the defense, but Parcells grew up on that side of the ball, so he could not completely divorce himself from it.

"When you have two geniuses, which they were, Bill Parcells being the established one and Belichick being the one on the way up at that point in time, some degree of friction is unavoidable. It's impossible, because they each have their own perspective of how they look at things," Martin said. "And, you know, it happened between Parcells and me, Parcells and Harry, Parcells and Phil, you can see videos of Parcells ripping Phil a new one because of a decision that Phil made in the heat of the game, that's to be expected. But that's not to say that creates a wedge between you and that individual for having a temporary different viewpoint on things."

Parcells received the Gatorade bath after each of the Giants' big victories in 1986. Following the NFC title game shutout of Washington, Belichick was lifted onto the shoulders of his defensive players and given a victory ride off the field. The photo appeared the next day on page one of the *New York Times*. Belichick saved as many copies as he could get his hands on.

Two weeks later, Parcells was given a victory ride off the field at the Rose Bowl.

One night they may even sit on the bench at Sea Girt and reminisce.

6

WHEN PHIL MET BILLY

Harry Burns (Billy Crystal) and his best friend Jess (Bruno Kirby) were sitting in the lower level of "Giants Stadium" watching Phil Simms drop back and complete a pass over the middle to tight end Mark Bavaro. The fans are cheering but Harry is distracted, depressed, and heartbroken. He's telling Jess that his wife Helen just blindsided him with news she not only wants a divorce but has already moved into a new apartment with her tax attorney boyfriend.

The life-changing revelation is taking place as Harry and Jess robotically join fans doing the wave and Harry is giving the painful details of the breakup and betrayal.

The conversation from the iconic romantic comedy *When Harry Met Sally* was actually filmed at a Buffalo Bills home game against the New England Patriots in 1988, but the action footage was from a Giants game against the Detroit Lions one week later at Giants Stadium. The producers staged the Crystal-Kirby scene at what was then known as Rich Stadium because the wave had not yet made its way to the Meadowlands.

It made perfect sense the game action involved the Giants. The movie was set in New York, Crystal's hometown, and he is a lifelong Giants fan. *When Harry Met Sally* may have publicly confirmed Crystal's devotion to Big Blue, but Simms already knew it. On January 23,

1987, two nights before they took on John Elway and the Denver Broncos in Super Bowl XXI at the Rose Bowl, Simms and teammate Phil McConkey found out Crystal was among the legion of woeful Giants fans who used to root for the downtrodden team to lose all their games toward the end of another dismal season, hoping to improve their draft position.

Not that it did any good.

The Giants arrived in Southern California on the Sunday before the Super Bowl and held their first practice of the week on Monday at the Los Angeles Rams facility in Anaheim. They spent the first of their two weeks of preparation back home in East Rutherford, which did not have an indoor practice field. After having practiced and played in bone-chilling weather the last three weeks of the regular season and the first two playoff games, the warm California air immediately rejuvenated their aching bones.

Simms's arm was alive. He was throwing fastballs and was amazingly sharp. He didn't want to peak too soon and leave his best throws on the practice field, but he felt great. There is no bigger stage in sports than the Super Bowl, especially for a New York quarterback with personality. It had been eighteen years since Joe Namath won Super Bowl III. Broadway Joe paraded around in fur coats, did pantyhose commercials and movies with Ann-Margret. Simms had a more conservative lifestyle than Namath, but the opportunities would be endless and lucrative if Simms played well enough to lead the Giants to their first Super Bowl victory. He tried to remain singularly focused on the game but received two enticing invitations. One was going to be fun, and the other was going to make him some money.

Disney was launching a brand-new high-profile ad campaign and requested that the winning quarterback—either Simms or Elway—recite the words that have since become synonymous with the Super Bowl MVP as he walks off the field: "I'm going to Disney World!" Simms was initially resistant to make plans based on winning the game—he thought that was a distraction, presumptuous, and bad luck and only gave in after Disney agreed to pay both quarterbacks the $50,000 fee regardless of the outcome. He was cognizant of Parcells having no patience for what the coach derisively called "celebrity quarterbacks."

David Fishof, a music producer and sports agent who represented Simms, had already set up a book deal for Simms and McConkey to be written by Dick Schaap, the highly respected author and television personality. Schaap had many influential friends, and he and Crystal met in January 1975 when Schaap was the editor of *Sport* magazine and Crystal was an unknown twenty-six-year-old comedian. Muhammad Ali was receiving the Sport Magazine Man of the Year at an awards dinner at the Plaza Hotel in Manhattan, and Schaap needed a comedian to perform. His first choice was the well-established Robert Klein, but he was not available. An agent from William Morris recommended Crystal. "Billy who?" was the reaction Schaap recounted in his book, *Before My Eyes*. The agent assured him Crystal was a funny guy. "He does a terrific imitation of Ali," she said. "Ali and Howard Cosell. You'll love him." Crystal was spectacular at the banquet, and his performance led him to become lifelong friends with Ali and Schaap. Crystal gave a memorable eulogy at Ali's funeral.

More than ten years after they first met, Crystal asked Schaap whether he could arrange a dinner for him with Simms and McConkey during Super Bowl week. Schaap set it for Friday night, after the Giants hardest practices and meetings were over for the week. Parcells moved the Giants out of the Westin South Coast Plaza Hotel in Costa Mesa after Friday's practice in Anaheim and bussed them to their new home at the Beverly Garland Hotel in North Hollywood for the last two nights before the game. The Garland sat next to the 101 freeway and was fourteen miles from the Rose Bowl in Pasadena. The Giants were now north of Los Angeles instead of south, which guaranteed a quicker game day trip to the stadium without having to deal with the suffocating LA traffic. Just as important, Parcells also didn't want the media, family, or superfans—known as "56-11s" for parading around in Taylor's and Simms's jerseys—knowing where his team was bunking the final forty-eight hours before kickoff. Parcells went all out to keep his players out of trouble. He even hired a security guard Super Bowl week to trail the troubled wide receiver Bobby Johnson twenty-four hours a day for seven days to make sure he wasn't meeting up with crack dealers. The Giants stayed away from scandal all week. No arrests. No bad headlines. In their free time, players went fishing or to the movies or out to dinner.

This much is certain: The Giants were aware there was no margin of error with Parcells. One screwup and they were on the first flight back to New Jersey. Aisle or window?

Simms and McConkey were the last two players Parcells had to worry about embarrassing the team on their Friday night off. Simms liked to watch TV in his room on the road. McConkey enjoyed partying back home, but even without any team-imposed in-season restrictions in New York, he had the self-imposed curfew. But nobody was going to be in a hurry to rush out of the restaurant on this Friday night. Rob Reiner, the director and coproducer of *When Harry Met Sally*, was a close friend of Crystal's and planned to join him, Simms, and McConkey but had to cancel at the last minute. It was Crystal, Simms, and McConkey eating seafood and talking football.

"Billy couldn't have been nicer," Simms said.

Maybe if Parcells knew the Giants offensive game plan was on the menu he wouldn't have let Simms and McConkey out of the hotel.

Crystal picked a spot close to the Beverly Garland. "We met at Orleans, a Cajun restaurant where everyone was eating spicy-hot blackened redfish Paul Prudhomme style," Crystal told me during the time he was in rehearsal in 2022 for his Broadway show, *Mr. Saturday Night*.

Near the end of dinner, Simms and McConkey gave the comedian access they were certain—and praying—would not come back to bite them, or even worse, make its way back to Parcells. Crystal, who was going to the Super Bowl, wanted the Giants to win the game, so he was not about to share inside information with Dan Reeves or Elway or anybody who stepped foot in the state of Colorado in the previous six months. Crystal was true blue.

It was not hard to imagine him turning this into one of his comedy routines.

"I asked Phil [Simms], if like the 49ers, they had the first twenty plays set. Phil said, 'Pretty much, but here's a few,'" Crystal said.

Crystal was wide eyed. Simms was about to take him inside the Super Bowl huddle.

"Well, here's what we're going to do," Simms told Crystal.

How much did he actually reveal?

"I told him about as much as I could give to a normal person, or to a person that wasn't in the game," Simms said as he briefly took over the storytelling of that night. "I told him the passes I was going to throw, how we were going to start the game, what I was going to do. And you know, he's like, 'Okay, really?' I said, 'Yeah, this is the very first play.'"

"Joe Morris was a great running back, and the Giants had a terrific sweep," Crystal said. "So, Phil says, 'Denver will be looking for that so we'll run that formation, but we'll fake [to Morris] and I'll hit Lionel Manuel down the middle for 22 yards.' Very specifically, 22 yards."

Game day at the Rose Bowl. Gorgeous weather in the mid-70s with the surrounding San Gabriel mountains providing a picturesque backdrop. The Beach Boys performed pregame. Neil Diamond sang a quick rendition of the national anthem and patted Parcells on the back as he jogged off the field. Parcells had his game face on for five hours already but still acknowledged Diamond, who is from Brooklyn. The Broncos were the visiting team and called the coin toss. Tom Jackson was one of five Broncos captains sent out to greet Harry Carson, the only one of New York's captains picked to represent the Giants. Co-captains George Martin and Simms remained on the sideline. The Giants were sending a message: Send the whole team out if you want. We're good with Harry and we're going to kick your ass.

Jackson and the Broncos won the coin toss and elected to receive the opening kickoff, and they picked up two first downs before the drive stalled at the Giants 31-yard line. Rich Karlis, one of both the best and last of the barefoot kickers in the NFL, came on to hit a 48-yard field goal, tying the longest in Super Bowl history. The Giants were already down 3–0, and Elway showed off the best arm in the NFL on the first drive.

The Giants first possession started at their 22 with 10:41 left in the first quarter. Crystal was sitting with his friends in the Rose Bowl. One of his buddies in particular came to believe Crystal was Mr. Football.

"So, I'm in the stands and the Giants come on the field to start their first drive, and the guy predicts the first play," Crystal said.

"Morris on a sweep," his friend said.

"Nope, Denver will be ready for that. So, Simms will fake it to him and hit Lionel Manuel for 22 yards down the middle," Crystal said.

"No way," his friend said.

"Twenty bucks?" Crystal said.

"You're on," his friend said.

Simms ran a play action fake to Morris, just as he told Crystal, and fired a 17-yard completion down the middle to Manuel. Simms was off in his prediction by five yards, but he won Crystal some money.

"I have to act cool but that's the first twenty bucks," Crystal said.

If Crystal was in the huddle, he would have looked at Simms and said, "You look mahvelous!"

Crystal's friend was shaking his head. He was bewildered. The Giants went against their season-long tendencies, and Crystal somehow got it right. If this was Wall Street, it's called insider trading. All of a sudden, he was not only Billy Crystal, he was John Madden.

"How did you know?" his friend said.

"I'm a big fan of the game. Make my own game plans," Crystal said.

Maybe so. Maybe not. Keep 'em guessing.

Parcells knew nothing of the dinner and certainly was not aware Simms's lips had become so loose. Simms's info would likely have been useless if the Giants had started the possession inside their 5-yard line. The ball would have gone to Morris to create breathing room.

"We knew we wanted to throw that pass early in the game, and the circumstances just happened to coincide with the game plan," Parcells said.

Can you imagine if Parcells, as protective and paranoid as any coach in NFL history, knew in advance that Simms was revealing the first play?

"No, I wouldn't have been happy," Parcells said.

He was not smiling.

Before the night was over, Crystal would score another victory off his friends. But first, there was more game to play.

═══

NEW YORK TRAILED 10–9 at the half, and it could have been worse. Denver had a first and goal at the Giants 1-yard line early in the second quarter, but an Elway scramble and two runs moved the Broncos back to the 6 before Karlis pushed a chip-shot 23-yard field goal wide right. Then with thirteen seconds left in the second quarter, he was wide right again, this time from 34 yards. The Giants, after scoring a touchdown early in the game on Simms's 6-yard pass to backup tight end Zeke Mowatt to take a 7–3 lead, fell behind 10–7 and moved within one point when Martin chased down Elway and sacked him in the end zone for a safety on a play that started from the Denver 13-yard line. In the Giants 19–16 victory over the Broncos during the 1986 regular season, Martin changed the game when he tipped Elway's screen pass, caught it himself, and took off on a 78-yard interception return, faking a lateral to Taylor along the way. He was finally brought down when Taylor jumped on his back in the end zone to celebrate. Parcells called it the greatest football play he's ever seen.

Parcells read his team perfectly coming out of the long Super Bowl "Salute to Hollywood's 100th Anniversary" halftime show and sensed they were energized despite the sluggish first half. "We were in a lackadaisical funk the first two quarters. What the fuck is going on?" Taylor said. "The best thing about Bill Parcells is any other coach would come in the locker room during halftime and be cussing us out and saying, 'Get your head out of your ass,' and all that shit. Parcells was cool. He walked in there and said, 'Okay. Everybody having fun? How about let's go out there and play some New York Giants football?' And

I said, 'We played two quarters, and we didn't play one down of New York Giants football.' Then we went out there and just tore ass."

The momentum flipped when the Giants faced a fourth and 1 from their own 46 on the opening possession of the third quarter. Parcells sent backup quarterback Jeff Rutledge in with the punt team and shifted into what he had named the "Arapahoe formation." Rutledge under center, running backs Lee Rouson and Maurice Carthon lined up in a split backfield, punter Sean Landeta five yards behind them. Rutledge kept the ball and pushed up the middle for two yards. First down. Parcells broke out a grin. It took guts for him to go for it on fourth down on the Giants' side of midfield still relatively early in a very close game.

He was not done with the tricks.

Simms finished off the drive by completing a 13-yard touchdown pass to Mark Bavaro with the Giants grabbing the lead for good, 16–10. They were just starting to roll. They held the Broncos to a three and out, and the Giants ended their next possession with Raul Allegre connecting on a 21-yard field goal for a 19–10 lead.

Parcells then made Crystal really look like Madden, who was calling the game with Pat Summerall on CBS. Denver again went three and out, and the Giants started at their 32. Morris ran for 2 yards, Simms hit Manuel for 17, and Morris ran for 4 yards. That moved New York to a second and 6 at the Denver 45 with less than a minute remaining in the third period.

As the Giants lined up, Crystal once again made a prediction to his friends. His mind went back to another moment at dinner. McConkey had used the salt-and-pepper shakers to diagram a trick play.

Crystal said McConkey told him, "We have a flea flicker we're gonna surprise them with. Phil hands it off, and Joe laterals it back, and I'll run a deep route and he'll hit me for 50–60 yards depending on where we are!"

Crystal already had twenty bucks in his pocket from the opening play. He decided this was a good time to play double or nothing.

"Watch for a flea flicker," he informed his friends. "Denver will never see it coming."

"Come on. The Giants don't run that kind of stuff!" his friend countered.

"Another twenty?" Crystal said.

"I got you this time," his friend said.

What happened next?

"Just like the salt shakers that McConkey moved near the crawfish, he grabs the pass for a huge gain. The guy thinks I'm a genius, and with my forty bucks I was able to buy two hot dogs and a beer!" Crystal said.

He was probably exaggerating. He could have bought at least one more beer. Game tickets for Super Bowl XXI cost only $75.

Just as McConkey had foretold, Simms took the snap, turned to his left, and tossed the ball to Morris. Little Joe then took a couple of steps toward the line of scrimmage, spun around, and with two hands flipped the ball back to Simms, who had retreated behind him. Simms dropped back two steps and then fired from his own 45 to McConkey, who was running right to left wide open through the Broncos secondary. Simms hit him in stride near the sideline at the Broncos 19. "I said at dinner it's going be helter-skelter in their defensive secondary, they're going to be caught off guard because it's so contra to anything we would do," McConkey said. "It was the most open I've ever been in my life at any level on a pass play. Even out on the street as a kid. Just to see their faces as I was cutting diagonally across the field, I could see linebackers, safeties, corners, when they realized that they had been tricked, and they were so out of position. I've never seen eyes get that big and mouths open like that. They knew they were caught, man. It's the most incredible feeling I think I've ever had on a football field."

McConkey could think of only one thing after Simms's perfect throw: fulfilling his dream of scoring a Super Bowl touchdown. He set his sights on the goal line as soon as he caught the pass. He tried to jump over cornerback Mark Haynes at the 5, got tripped up and did a complete somersault, and landed 1 yard short of the end zone for a 44-yard gain, the Giants' longest play of the day. McConkey wound up face down in the end zone banging his fists into the Rose Bowl grass. "The emotions were so mixed realizing it was a huge play, knowing we were going to score probably the game-clinching play," McConkey said. "So, I'm kind of elated. But at the same time, extremely frustrated that I was that close to something I dreamed about my whole life. I always talked about it. And, you know, I didn't score too many touchdowns in the NFL, and I told Simms I'm going to score a touchdown in the Super Bowl."

Haynes was a former teammate of McConkey's, and they battled each other in practice for two years. He was the Giants first-round pick in 1980 and played six years in New York before Parcells traded him to the Broncos in April 1986 for two second-round picks and a sixth-round pick. He went to the University of Colorado, never seemed to enjoy New York, was happy to be in Denver, and would have loved to get revenge on his former team. "Mark Haynes was a pretty good player, but he was a sour little son of a bitch," Parcells said.

Morris scored on the next play after the flea flicker to give the Giants a 26–10 lead twenty-four seconds into the fourth quarter. The game was all but over, but Parcells scolded Rouson and rookie Pepper Johnson on the sideline for celebrating prematurely even though it would have taken the biggest comeback in Super Bowl history for the Giants to lose this game.

McConkey made his touchdown prediction come true the next time the Giants had the ball on a pass that bounced off the facemask of Bavaro, the godfather of his daughter, who followed in her father's footsteps and attended the Naval Academy.

Almost twenty years after Super Bowl XXI, Simms had a chance to see Crystal perform in person in his one-man Broadway show *700 Sundays* at the Broadhurst Theatre on Forty-Fourth Street. He went with his younger son Matt, a nephew, and an eighty-year-old friend. "It was maybe the best Broadway play I ever went to, and I went to a lot,"

Simms said. He sat in a balcony box relatively close to the stage. "It was hilarious," he said. "I was exhausted from laughing."

It was Crystal's way of paying him back after Simms won him a couple of hot dogs, a beer, and a lot of respect.

———

PARCELLS WAS HAPPY with the Giants' preparation during Super Bowl week and canceled the Saturday walk-through. The linebackers went over to the Rose Bowl and changed into Superman costumes to pose for a United Way charity poster. Simms never got much sleep the night before games. Super Bowl Eve was no different. "I wasn't nervous," he said. "I like to sit there and watch TV and relax."

Simms's Saturday night started by going to the movies with McConkey and Bavaro to see *Platoon*, then he retired to his room and put on *Saturday Night Live*. The guest host was Joe Montana. The last time Simms saw Joe Cool was a few weeks earlier in the divisional round of the playoffs, won by the Giants 49–3, when Jim Burt blasted Montana with a vicious but legal hit. Montana was the fourth quarterback the '86 Giants knocked out of a game. Simms and Montana were bitter rivals, fueled by San Francisco coach Bill Walsh making it clear that he had Simms ranked ahead of Montana as the best quarterback in the 1979 draft.

Montana led Simms 2–0 in Super Bowl victories, but Simms led him 2–1 in head-to-head playoff matchups, and now he was less than twenty-hours from his chance to not only close the Super Bowl gap on Montana but carve a place for himself in NFL history. It was funny that watching Montana on *SNL* helped keep him calm. "When they got done, I said, 'Damn, Joe's pretty good,'" Simms said.

After their careers ended, Simms and Montana became good friends. Simms and his son Matt run a quarterback school in New Jersey, and Montana called Phil and asked whether he would work with his younger son Nick, a college quarterback. Joe was frustrated because Nick wasn't accepting his advice and thought it would be better to take a step back and have Simms do the instructing.

While Nick was with Simms getting in productive work, Joe and his wife Jennifer were on a luxurious European vacation.

"Call your dad," Phil said to Nick after one of the workouts.

Nick called. Joe answered. Nick handed his phone to Phil.

"Here I am throwing with your son and you're on some damn yacht cruising around Italy on the Riviera," Simms said.

They shared a good laugh.

Simms was able to sleep for a couple of hours the night before the Super Bowl and was in the lobby early to take a taxi to the Rose Bowl. He rode with two of his starting offensive linemen, left tackle Brad Benson and right guard Chris Godfrey, which had been the routine all season. Parcells was happy game day had finally arrived. On the day after the NFC Championship Game victory against Washington, he had ninety-nine ticket requests from family, current friends, and college friends he hadn't heard from in forever. He had a clause in his contract that allowed him to buy an allotment of tickets, but he ran right through those, and Giants co-owner Tim Mara—he and Parcells were very close—supplied him with the rest. Simms bought twenty-six tickets at $75 each for family and friends.

All season, Parcells and trainer Ronnie Barnes took a taxi together to the stadium. "We had a rule. On the curb at 7:30," Parcells said. He wasn't about to change things on the morning of the biggest game of his life. Parcells is so superstitious that if a black cat crossed in front of him when he was driving, he felt compelled to put the car in reverse to where the feline had the nerve to appear in order to erase the jinx. He collected statues of elephants, but only if the trunks pointed up. Before he and Barnes got in the taxi, they had breakfast together.

"One funny thing happened in the coffee shop," Parcells said. "I was kind of quiet. I wasn't saying much. And so Ronnie says to me, 'What's the matter with you?' I said to him, 'I'm just worried about Elway a little bit.'" Barnes is a soft-spoken man from North Carolina who had been with the Giants since 1976. He was fired up for the game. "He gets loud and says, 'We're going to chase that son of a bitch out to the parking lot.' That kind of calmed me down a little bit."

Kickoff wasn't until 3:13 p.m. PT, but Parcells and Barnes were in the taxi at 7:45 a.m. and inside the stadium by 8:15 a.m. Parcells was walking the field before nine trying to come up with any edge he could pass on to his players. He bumped into George Toma, brought in by the NFL every year to prepare the Super Bowl field. Toma told him the field was a little oily and the back of the end zone was very close to the stands. "He said the receivers have to be careful down there," Parcells said. Starting safety Herb Welch joined the Giants as a rookie in 1985 from UCLA, which moved its home games from the Los Angeles Coliseum to the Rose Bowl beginning in 1982. Welch shared his insight on the stadium with Parcells.

The Giants home team locker room was small, but at least it was bigger than training camp at Pace, which was so bad Simms said it made his locker room at Southern High School in Louisville and little Morehead State in Kentucky look like the Taj Mahal. By the time the players arrived at the Rose Bowl, though, equipment bags were laid out in the middle of the room, and it was cramped, with no space to walk around for coaches and players. Parcells had a pregame issue that was bugging him. NFL rules dictate that any player not dressed for the Super Bowl had to sit in the stands. They were prohibited from watching from the sidelines, the usual vantage point for inactive and injured players. Parcells didn't like that rule. He knew even if they weren't in uniform, each of the players had contributed in some way and deserved to be on the sidelines. Parcells found a security guard the NFL hired for the game, who happened to be from Yonkers just outside New York City.

"I said if you see them take the players off the field, you let them back on," Parcells said.

He opened his wallet and handed the guy $100.

"I don't want to worry about this," Parcells said.

"Don't worry," the guard said.

As with most things that season, Parcells got his way.

——

SIMMS WAS THE most underrated and unappreciated quarterback of his era. Even Parcells dumped on him when he was promoted to replace Ray Perkins in 1983. He chose Scott Brunner, who led the Giants to the playoffs in 1981 after Simms was injured, to start the season opener. Parcells came to the Giants in 1981, and Simms suffered a season-ending separated shoulder in mid-November. Then he suffered season-ending torn right knee ligaments in the 1982 Giants–Jets preseason game when he was hit by Joe Klecko and Abdul Salaam. Parcells had not seen much of Simms on the field and went with the less talented but more familiar Brunner to open the season. Simms immediately demanded a trade. The Giants refused.

When Parcells broke the news to Simms that he would begin the season on the bench, it didn't surprise him. He thought the assistant coaches were supporting him but knew Parcells was not. Simms was the Giants' first-round pick after George Young became general manager in 1979, had suffered through a series of unfortunate injuries, and now was being told that he was beaten out by Brunner, a sixth-round pick from Delaware in 1980. It was a conversation that has remained in Simms's memory for decades.

"Here's what I'm going to do. I'm going with Scott Brunner and you're going to be the backup. You got any problems with that?" Parcells said.

"Fuck it, of course I do. I got a lot of problems with it," Simms said. "You can trade me. I don't care. I would love to leave."

He left the room, called his agent, and told him to get him out of New York. "I'm sure Bill wanted to trade me just because he didn't want to put up with this guy," Simms said. "But those feelings changed pretty quick. Even that year, I could already feel he wanted to go back to me early."

Brunner struggled in the Giants 2–3 start, Parcells switched to Simms during the sixth game, and on his third series, his season ended when he suffered a grotesque injury to his thumb after hitting it on the helmet of Eagles defensive end Carl Hairston. "When he finally put me in, I got hurt. It's unbelievable," Simms said. The Giants finished 3–12–1, and Simms believes if he had been the quarterback and the season still spiraled out of control, the Giants would have dumped him as one of the many roster casualties.

After the season, the Giants traded Brunner to Denver, seemingly sold on Simms going forward. But first they brought in free agent quarterback Warren Moon of the Canadian Football League for a visit. Moon elected to sign with the Houston Oilers, and the Giants set up a training camp competition between Simms and Jeff Rutledge that was more for show. Rutledge was a ninth-round pick in Simms's draft in 1979 and was acquired during the preseason in 1982 after Simms suffered his knee injury. Simms easily won the job and became the first Giants quarterback to throw for 4,000 yards in a season in 1984, and he led them to the second round of the playoffs in 1984 and 1985. By then, Simms had become one of Parcells's favorites.

"We came to an understanding after the 1983 season that both our careers are going to be on the line the following year," Simms said. "And his exact words were, 'Simms, if I ever survive this, by God, we're going to do it my way.' He was a different guy in training camp that year. He was all over it. I knew he was behind me."

That didn't earn him any favors. No player was coached harder by Parcells than Simms, but no player improved more, either. Parcells worked hard to keep his players on edge. He believed insecurity brought out their best. "There is always a crisis, and whose turn was it going to be today? I hated it when it was me," Simms said. "It was really a tension-filled day. I would come home exhausted from the tension. Practice was real. I got nervous before the seven on sevens. I got nervous before the team drills. I knew the performance had to be good. No exaggeration, just a fact. That was his MO. He loved friction. If it wasn't there, he created it. A lot of times, I was the perfect foil."

Parcells's methods didn't work with everybody. But it worked with Simms and culminated in the Super Bowl, where he was nearly perfect, completing twenty-two of twenty-five passes for 268 yards, with three touchdowns and no interceptions. His 88 percent completion rate remains an NFL postseason record. He was ten for ten in the second half. It came following a regular season when he threw more interceptions (twenty-two) than touchdowns (twenty-one). It finished off an odd postseason for Simms. In the lopsided victory against the 49ers, he had only nine completions, but four of them went for touchdowns. He had only seven completions in the championship game against Washington.

Parcells never cared about Simms's numbers. His standard for measuring quarterbacks was whether he got his team in the end zone. As they walked out of the locker room at Giants Stadium for the 1984 season opener, Parcells told Simms if he didn't throw two interceptions, it meant he wasn't taking enough chances. He didn't want his quarterback playing scared. Simms didn't throw any interceptions that day against the Eagles in a 28–27 victory, but he did throw four touchdowns, and his 409 yards passing was the jumping-off point for the Giants becoming playoff contenders.

"Bill was really tough. For real. He was tough," Simms said. "And it helped us win. It was the main driving force. But it causes a lot of friction too. When we all get away from it, and it's all over, we all sit around and go, 'Man, thank God, he changed our lives.'"

Parcells and Simms had a famous blowup on the sidelines in Indianapolis that was caught on camera during a Monday night game in 1990. They had a relationship that allowed them to yell at each other and laugh about it later. Simms refused to back down, and that earned him even more respect from teammates who would have loved to yell at Parcells but didn't have the job security to take that risk. Parcells was so competitive and such a perfectionist that no matter the game or the score, he didn't let up.

Simms was having a Super Bowl that kids dream about when they are throwing passes in their backyard. Nothing hits the dirt. Every pass has zip and is on the money. Receivers are covered, but the ball finds the tightest window. Simms was in that zone in Pasadena. He went through the game and didn't make any mistakes. Phil's experience with his father William prepared him to play for Parcells. William never coached Phil in any sport and sadly was short on praise. Phil rushed home from a youth baseball game anxious to tell his dad he pitched a no-hitter and hit three home runs.

Dad's reaction to the no-hitter:

"You didn't throw too many curveballs, did you?"

His reaction to the three home runs:

"Yeah? Did you hit them or did you pop them up?"

William had taken all the joy out of Phil's day. "By the time he got done, I felt like I failed," Simms said.

On Super Bowl Sunday, Simms had the equivalent of a no-hitter with three home runs, and even with Parcells playing the part of William Simms, nobody was taking the joy out of being the Super Bowl MVP. Not that Parcells didn't try. The Giants were up 26–10 with ten minutes left. They had a second and goal at the Broncos 1-yard line looking to add on. Simms took a 5-yard sack and on the next play threw the pass that bounced off Bavaro's facemask in the end zone right to McConkey's anxious arms to put the game away. The Giants were up 33–10, but Parcells reacted like they were down 33–10 when Simms reached the sideline. He got all over him for taking the sack.

"Oh, come on, give me a break!" Simms shouted. "I don't want to hear it. The coaching lessons are over for today."

The next time the Giants had the ball, they scored on a 2-yard run by Ottis Anderson. New York scored on its first five possessions of the second half. Even Parcells was smiling at the end.

═══

AS SOON AS Broncos backup quarterback Gary Kubiak was sacked by Giants rookie defensive end Eric Dorsey on the final play of Super Bowl XXI, Simms started to walk across the field to seek out Elway. He got a tap on the shoulder.

"Hey, Phil, don't forget Disney World," a Disney representative said.

"Oh God, what do you want me to do?" Simms said.

After he said yes to Fishof on Friday night, Simms put Mickey and Minnie out of his mind. "I said yes to get everybody to shut up," he said. He was caught up in the emotion of winning the Super Bowl and Super Bowl MVP and had to be reminded of his line.

The commercial opened with, "Phil Simms, you've just won the Super Bowl. What are you doing next?"

"I'm going to go to Disney World!" for the East Coast audience.

"I'm going to go to Disneyland!" for the West Coast audience.

He did five takes for each. He started on the sidelines and was done before he reached midfield. With the song "When You Wish upon a Star" as the background music, the commercial showed highlights of Simms from the Super Bowl and then cuts to him saying the now-famous words. In the time it took to recite his lines, Simms missed meeting Elway at midfield.

He fought the Disney proposal for days, but decades later, he takes pride in being the first Disney Super Bowl star. "Players don't mind doing it now," he said. "They see what it brings and the whole thing is kind of cool."

Even though the Super Bowl was played in Southern California and Disneyland is in Anaheim just south of Los Angeles, Simms did not go straight to the theme park, which is now part of the tradition after taping the commercial. He traveled home with the Giants the day after the game for the victory parade on Tuesday. New York mayor Ed Koch refused to give the champs the traditional ticker tape parade down the Canyon of Heroes in lower Manhattan because the team moved to New Jersey in 1976. The Giants instead held their celebration at Giants Stadium. Koch was in Warsaw, Poland.

When the '86 Giants recall how Koch turned his back on them, it is usually followed by a few expletives. They still resent him depriving them of one of the greatest experiences of winning a championship as a New York team. Right after the parade in the stadium, Simms was back on a plane to Los Angeles to make an appearance on *The Tonight Show*. Before he left New Jersey, the talent booker told Simms that

Johnny Carson, the legendary host, was off that week. They gave him the option to wait until Carson returned the following week or do the show with guest host Garry Shandling.

He elected to appear with Shandling. "I really liked him," Simms said. "I loved the show."

Next up was receiving the Super Bowl MVP car and then taking his family to Disney World in Orlando later in the offseason with a visit to Space Mountain, his favorite ride. It was a whirlwind for a kid from Kentucky from a family of eight children that never had much. They lived on his grandfather's tobacco farm in Springfield, Kentucky, until his parents bought a small house in Louisville, where the five boys slept in one bedroom and the three girls slept in another.

He was lying in bed the night after the Super Bowl watching television with his wife, Diana, at their home in New Jersey. "We saw the commercial," he said. "We couldn't believe it. That was really, really unbelievable."

When he bumped into friends, the conversation was not about his record-setting performance. "It was amazing. Everybody wanted to talk about the Disney commercial," Simms said. "What about the game?"

The commercial was so well received that Disney has not changed the format. It's almost always the Super Bowl MVP, with a few exceptions.

"I think it's really cool that I was the first," Simms said. "It's a trivia question."

———

SIMMS IS ONE of the life-after-football success stories of the '86 Giants. He became the first big-name casualty of the salary cap era when the Giants cut him one month before training camp in 1994. He was coming off surgery on March 1 to repair a torn labrum in his throwing shoulder after leading the Giants to an 11–5 record and their first playoff spot in the post-Parcells era. They came within one game of winning the NFC East and earning the No. 1 seed in the NFC but

lost a thrilling overtime game to Dallas in the final week of the regular season at Giants Stadium. Instead of receiving a first-round bye,
they defeated the Vikings in the wild-card game but were humiliated
by the 49ers in the divisional round, losing 44–3 in San Francisco in
what turned out to be the final game in the careers of Simms and Taylor. Simms was working out in the weight room at Giants Stadium in
mid-June, rehabbing his shoulder, when he was summoned to coach
Dan Reeves's office. Reeves was the Broncos coach seven years earlier
against the Giants in the Super Bowl and had just completed his first
season in New York.

Simms took the elevator up one level to the Giants executive
offices. He was due to make a career-high $2.5 million in 1994 and was
ten weeks removed from surgery. It was the first year of the salary cap
system. Reeves loved Simms. The prospect of getting released didn't
cross Simms's mind as they sat down to talk. Simms actually thought
Reeves had asked him to come up to sign some footballs for a charity
event. Instead, he was given the option to retire or be released.

Simms believed he could still play and wasn't prepared to call it
quits. He was thirty-eight years old, had missed almost two complete
seasons earlier in his career, and still was making up for lost time. He
was ready to play. When the Giants hired Young, they gave him total
control of football operations, and Wellington Mara never interfered
on player personnel matters. Young's decision to draft Simms as a
rookie GM was widely panned. NFL fans were not as savvy about the
draft as they are now when they are educated about the backup left
tackle from Idaho State or the starting safety from Boise State. They
had no clue who this Simms guy was. The Giants fans at the Waldorf
Astoria loudly booed the pick after Pete Rozelle announced it. NFL
Films was caught off guard and wanted to capture the moment and
asked Rozelle to announce the pick a second time, which gave the
fans the opportunity to boo a second time. Rozelle did it with a grin
on his face.

"Rozelle may have thought it was funny," Simms said. "I thought
it was the wrong thing for him to do."

The night before the draft, Young was sitting in his office with Mara and Perkins finalizing the decision to draft Simms. "If we pick Phil Simms, you're going to have to build barricades by the Lincoln Tunnel because the mobs are going to be after us," Mara said. "I'm all for it if you think he's the best man for the job."

Fifteen years later, Young made the decision to cut Simms, with Reeves given the job of delivering the message. Mara may not have agreed with all of Young's moves over the years, but he never publicly questioned one.

Until June 15, 1994.

"This is a day of overwhelming sadness for me," Mara said.

Mara didn't want Simms cut, but his loyalty to long-standing Giants players, coaches, and staff contributed to the darkest period of the franchise, when they failed to make the playoffs for nearly two decades. Young resurrected the Giants, and Mara didn't have it in him to reject his decision even though most around the team believed Simms could still play and was certainly still better than youngsters Dave Brown and Kent Graham.

Simms was hired by ESPN to work in the studio, but he still had the itch to play. He nearly signed to play for Buddy Ryan and the Arizona Cardinals in late September, but they couldn't agree on the money. The following March, he met with Bill Belichick, who was entering his fourth season as the Browns' coach, at a New Jersey hotel. Belichick wanted Simms to come in to back up Vinny Testaverde. Simms took a private plane to Cleveland with the intent to sign. The Browns had a press conference set up, but again, Simms couldn't reach agreement on a contract.

Tom Coughlin, the former Giants receivers coach, called to offer Simms the opportunity to play for his expansion Jacksonville Jaguars, who were beginning play in 1995. Coughlin wanted a veteran to help establish his disciplined culture in a locker room that was going to be dominated by young players. Simms and Coughlin each learned from Parcells what was required to win in the NFL, but Simms said thanks but no thanks.

The most intriguing possibility for Simms was discussed in the Giants Stadium parking lot after the Giants lost to the Cowboys in the 1993 regular season finale. Simms was walking up the ramp behind the west end zone on his way to his car in the players' parking lot. The Cowboys' three team buses were parked on the ramp, loading up for the trip to Newark Airport and the flight back to Dallas.

Simms admired the job Jimmy Johnson had done in Dallas after taking over for Tom Landry in 1989, improving from 1–15 in his first season to winning the Super Bowl in his fourth year, and he was now three victories away from repeating. Simms thought he had maybe one more year left with the Giants after Young drafted Brown in the first round of the 1992 supplemental draft.

The Cowboys had future Hall of Famer Troy Aikman at quarterback, but Simms had thought finishing his career in Dallas playing for Johnson and backing up Aikman could be an appealing option. He saw Johnson standing by one of the Cowboys buses and approached him.

"I want to play for you when I'm done here," Simms told Johnson.

Johnson had brought in veteran Bernie Kosar, his former quarterback at the University of Miami, during the season after he was cut by the Browns. Kosar signed with the Dolphins in 1994, so the Cowboys would have had an opening.

Simms never had a chance to follow up.

Four weeks later, the Cowboys won the Super Bowl again. In late March, Dallas owner Jerry Jones paid Johnson $2 million to leave the Cowboys in the highest-profile divorce in NFL history. When the Giants cut Simms ten weeks later, playing for Johnson in Dallas was no longer an option. If Johnson had remained, Simms very well could have been wearing the helmet with the star. Johnson didn't specifically recall the conversation with Simms in the excitement after winning the game against the Giants, but he indicated it would have been a logical move. "I always wanted three quarterbacks," he said. "The starter. A veteran at number two. A young future at number three. Phil would have fit right in."

Mara wanted to retire Simms's jersey No. 11 in 1994, but he wasn't ready. He was still bitter about the way he was let go and was holding out hope he could resume his career. He agreed in 1995, after the Browns deal fell through, to let the Giants retire his jersey at halftime of their season opener against Dallas. Simms ended his speech by declaring he had two wishes. The first was to run out on the field in front of the fans at Giants Stadium one more time. He had just done that.

"And lastly, for my second wish, I wanted to throw one more pass in my Giants jersey," he said. "So, who better to catch that pass than the greatest Giants player of all time, Lawrence Taylor."

Taylor was wearing a sports jacket, dress slacks, dress shoes, and a baseball cap. Simms sent him out twenty yards and lobbed a pass into his waiting arms. The crowd went wild. Taylor ran back to an approaching Simms, and the two icons of the '86 Giants shared an emotional embrace with Taylor kissing Simms on the cheek. The event provided Simms with closure.

He left ESPN to join NBC's number-one team broadcasting AFC games in 1995 and jumped to CBS's number-one team in 1998 when the network acquired the AFC rights. He remained on the number-one team until he was replaced by former Cowboys quarterback Tony Romo in 2017. CBS moved him to *The NFL Today* studio show. Although he would rather have left the booth on his terms, he knew that driving to the CBS studios on Fifty-Seventh Street and Eleventh Avenue in Manhattan would be a lot less physically demanding, and he had reached the point where that was important.

In the volatile world of network television, Simms has lived a charmed life. Off the field, he has dealt with real-life health problems including a back issue that was overwhelming. "When you get out of football you have to go right into preservation mode," he said. "If you play a long time, respect it."

Financially, life after football has been lucrative. In addition to the television work, he has numerous endorsements. Physically, life after football has at times been debilitating. It's not about showing symptoms of CTE, although he took plenty of big hits, especially early in his career when the Giants offensive line could not protect him.

It's about the rest of his body.

Simms is fair-skinned and from head to toe has been treated for skin cancer. He liked to play tennis and was a scratch golfer, and all those hot summer days on the practice field caught up to him. He's been forced to give up most outdoor activities, including golf, and wears sunscreen on every exposed area of his body whenever he's in the sun. He even puts lotion under his socks to protect his ankles. Doctors have told him he has no resistance to the sun.

"Any part of my body that has seen the sun has got an issue," Simms said. "Any place that I had exposed to the sun is in trouble. The only thing I didn't expose was my ass and whatever. That's it. I never did that. Thank God."

Simms is mentally sharp and still performing well on national television. But he absorbed some vicious hits in his career. As he was throwing a 15-yard touchdown pass to Bobby Johnson in the final minutes of the first half in the 49–3 victory over the 49ers in the '86 playoffs, Simms was hit so hard he heard a San Francisco defender say, "I killed him." Jim Burt and Taylor came off the sideline to hold him up and get him off the field. "Did we get a touchdown?" he asked Burt.

The Giants next possession came in the third quarter. Simms was at quarterback. Even now, he's still searching for answers how the play resulted in a touchdown.

"I don't know how it got there," Simms said. "I got hit in the mouth and lost a little chip off a tooth." Two plays later, Burt sent Joe Montana to the hospital with a concussion.

In the season opener the next year in Chicago, Simms was fuzzy after taking a big hit from Richard Dent on a pass intended for Lionel Manuel. Jeff Rutledge replaced him for one play, and Simms came back in to complete the series.

"Sixty-six 336 Y Cross," he called in the huddle.

When he came to the sideline, Parcells could tell something was off. "What's wrong?" he asked.

"I called a play and had no idea what it meant," Simms told him.

Rutledge finished out the second quarter. Simms collected himself at halftime and was back in.

Simms and Montana played in an era where it was open season on quarterbacks. They took brutal hits that today draw fifteen-yard penalty flags. The rules have changed to keep quarterbacks in the game by reducing the standard for roughing the passer and as a result reducing the big hits. That in part allowed Tom Brady to play twenty-three seasons and retire relatively unscathed. "If you hit somebody now, you get thrown out of the game," Taylor said. "I wouldn't have a check at the end of the game." Montana has endured more than two dozen surgeries since he retired after the 1994 season, including three neck fusions.

Simms was a workout warrior during his fifteen-year career. The combination of lifting weights at the stadium in the offseason after running two miles in the morning, and the torque of throwing a football took a tremendous toll on his back. When his career was over, he put stress on his back as a scratch golfer and playing tennis. He discovered after his playing days that he had spinal stenosis, a condition that puts pressure on the spinal cord, the nerves in the spine, and results in neck and back pain. Simms said he was born with stenosis but didn't know he had it until he was in his early fifties. He would do stretching exercises, work with foam rollers, work out a little bit. The relief he felt was short-lived. Twenty minutes. Simms was out of football twenty years and already had three back surgeries. "I had a discectomy. I had a little chip in one of my discs and then I had two for stenosis," Simms said. "They weren't bad."

The pain kept returning. The 2014 season doing games for CBS was torture. He was in so much pain. Walking through airports was a chore. Fifty feet seemed like fifty miles. He had to stop every twenty minutes in the terminal to wipe the sweat pouring down his face from the pain. If he bent down as if to tie his shoes, he would get temporary relief. Planes, car services, hotels, three hours broadcasting a game, and then reversing the travel to get back home, he feared his broadcasting career was in jeopardy. His body couldn't handle it. "It was brutal," he said. "The surgery had just shut my body down so bad. When the muscles shut down, it causes pain. Nothing worked. Many nights I would literally just walk around, go sit down, watch TV for twenty minutes, get up, walk around the house and stay up the whole night. Never sleep one second, many, many, many nights."

In the summer of 2015, he went to a Giants preseason contest at MetLife Stadium specifically to meet with Dr. Warren, the long-time team doctor. "I was so miserable, I didn't know what I was going to do," he said.

He arrived at the stadium, and the Giants doctors asked him to touch his toes and do some squats. He was flexible, but everything he tried hurt. Simms said Warren and the other doctors wanted to do some more tests in New York. But the regular season was approaching, and Simms had a preseason game for CBS the next weekend in San Diego. The pain was so bad that it felt to Simms like it was a matter of survival. "Doc Warren, who I trust and has done so much for me, wanted me to find a way to get through the season," Simms said. "Then we would really do some work." Simms needed more immediate help but knew he couldn't find time in his schedule with the season weeks away to fully treat his back pain. He was resigned to heading back to the broadcast booth still hurting. He was miserable missing games as a player. He did not miss any games as a broadcaster.

Simms left the stadium before the kickoff of the Giants preseason game. He was depressed. "I walked out of there and went, 'I got no answers.' That's when I freaked out," he said. "Fuck me. I got to live with this."

The twenty-mile drive home to Franklin Lakes gave him time to assess his physical and mental state. He parked out front of his ten-thousand-square-foot home, which sits on twenty acres, with a lake on the property. He walked through the front door into his family room and put the Giants game on television. He was so uncomfortable. He got down on the floor and raised his knees to his chest trying to reduce the pain. That didn't work.

Then he went to the cabinet where he keeps his liquor and took out a bottle of vodka. He filled a good-sized glass nearly to the top and chugged it in two gulps. Then he filled up a second glass and chugged that one, too. "I was truly drinking a glass of vodka like it was water. I was trying to numb the pain," he said. As he described the night, he said, "I was taking something else, too." He doesn't remember the name of the painkillers he swallowed while he was drinking the vodka, but the pain persisted.

The combination of alcohol and painkillers is not recommended. "No shit," he said. "But it didn't do anything. I didn't even get drunk. My body was just on fire. So, I drink it just trying to relax and I couldn't even relax. Oh my God, oh my God."

Simms is a social drinker. Mixing vodka and painkillers was out of desperation, not habit. His father, William, was an alcoholic. He would drink around the clock for five days straight and then be sober for two months. Even though alcoholism was in his family, Simms was not worried about becoming dependent on alcohol to relieve his pain.

"I never thought about that because I knew I could control it. I wasn't a drinker," he said.

How many times did he do the vodka-painkiller combination?

"It was just a short period," Simms said.

He paused.

"Yeah, it wasn't long," he said.

It was at that very point, lying on the floor with a glass of vodka and a bottle of painkillers by his side, that he felt his career doing games on television was over. "I was in that much misery," he said.

He thought he was doomed to be one of the long list of former players who went through the rest of their lives in pain. From the fetal position in his family room, Simms called his son Chris, who had experience with pain management.

Chris narrowly avoided dying on the field when he played for the Bucs in 2006 after his spleen ruptured in the third game of the season against the Panthers in Tampa, possibly from a hit in the first quarter. It was initially thought to be bruised ribs. He was also suffering from dehydration, and after getting fluids in the locker room, he insisted on coming back in and led a fourth-quarter rally that nearly won the game. It was determined after the game that he was bleeding internally, and he was rushed to St. Joseph's Hospital a few blocks from Raymond James Stadium to have his spleen removed. Phil had just landed in Newark after doing a game in Pittsburgh when he got the news about Chris. He didn't leave the airport and flew right to Tampa.

The injury ended Chris Simms's season and all but ended his career. He never played another snap for the Bucs. He spent most of 2007 on injured reserve in Tampa and was with the Titans in 2008 and 2010 and the Broncos in 2009. He attempted a total of just six passes after the spleen injury. When he was in Denver, he discovered Greg Roskopf, the founder of Muscle Activation Techniques. He helped Chris in his one season with the Broncos. Phil had visited him once on Chris's recommendation. When Phil called Chris as he was downing the painkillers and chasing them with vodka, his son implored him to see Roskopf again. His back had gotten much worse than the first time he visited him.

"He knows how the body works," Phil Simms said. "If your left arm hurts, maybe it's because your right shoulder is tight. It's hard to explain, but it's muscle activation."

First, he had to go to San Diego to broadcast a Chargers preseason game. When he landed, he called Mike Carey, the former NFL referee who at the time was working for CBS as its rules analyst. His daughter was a wellness consultant, and Simms immediately went to see her. She helped him get through the weekend. On the way home, he stopped off in Denver to see Roskopf and stayed for three or four days.

"He would work on me and fix me and tell me what was going on in my body," he said. When he first arrived, Roskopf had Simms extend his arm, and he couldn't resist the weight of Roskopf pushing down with his finger. By the time he left, Simms was doing so much better, he felt he could resist the weight of a truck on his arm. "He did it to my whole body," he said. He went back to see Roskopf a half-dozen times during the 2015 season on his way home from West Coast games and has since sent friends to Denver to see him.

"That's who saved my life," Simms said. "He fixed me and gave me a chance."

———

MCCONKEY DIDN'T HAVE enough salt-and-pepper shakers at dinner with Billy Crystal to diagram the final play in Super Bowl XXI. Besides, even Billy wouldn't have bet on it.

As the final seconds ticked off the clock of the Giants' victory, Harry Carson snuck up behind Parcells and dumped a bucket of Gatorade on his head. Jim Burt grabbed his young son out of the Rose Bowl stands and carried him around on his shoulders. Then when the game was over, Simms did the Disney commercial, Parcells was carried off the field, and Pepper Johnson and Williams Roberts, teammates at Ohio State and now Super Bowl champions, went to the middle of the field, put down their helmets, and danced.

In the weeks after the game, Simms and his family went to the Magic Kingdom, all expenses paid by Disney. It was an ending fit for a champion.

PART III

AFTER THE CONFETTI

7

HANDS DOWN

B obby Johnson's life story is told by his hands.

Together they produced the most memorable catch in the Giants' journey to the Super Bowl in 1986. It came on fourth and 17 with just over one minute remaining, on the road against Minnesota, trailing by a point. Johnson hauled in a terrific sideline pass from Simms, picking up the first down and anchoring a drive that ended in a game-winning field goal. It was a simple catch, Johnson clutching a well-placed ball to his chest and stepping out of bounds to stop the clock. It was a turning point. Johnson's hands snatched victory away from the Vikings. And the Giants did not lose again the rest of the season.

Individually, Johnson's hands each relay their own dramatic story.

The left hand is where Johnson wears his prized possession, the Super Bowl XXI ring, and it represents how many self-imposed obstacles he's overcome in his tragic journey. He once sold it to a pawn shop in Nashville for $450 to pay for his crack addiction and a fleabag $29 hotel room to briefly avoid both sleeping on a park bench and going hungry. Johnson's left hand remained bare for almost thirty years.

The right hand is grossly disfigured after it was sucked into a powerful pencil manufacturing machine at his job eight years after the

Super Bowl and lost half its pinky and ring and middle fingers in the accident. He looks at that hand, tearfully recalls his catch in Minnesota, and reminds himself it helped cradle Simms's pass.

Johnson is a friendly guy with an outgoing personality and is once again popular among the '86 crew after ostracizing himself for many years with his drug use. He is grateful to be alive after nearly jumping off a bridge one night into the freezing cold Cumberland River in the late '90s. He survived that moment of despair, so he is not embarrassed by the grotesque appearance of his right hand, salvaged by skin grafts from his thigh and stomach. His right hand looks like a slab of meat when he offers it in a handshake.

"My hands," he said. "That was my pride."

He lifted up his shirt to reveal a large scar on his stomach. In order for the graft to take hold, "my hand was sewed to my stomach for two months," he said.

Johnson has come to embrace his right hand as part of who he is. The left hand was rewarded by the return of his Super Bowl ring three decades after the right hand was punished by his desperate need for money after drugs ended his promising career following the Super Bowl season. He made $400,000 in three years with the Giants before taxes and estimates he spent $40,000 on crack.

"Almost every one of the guys on that '86 team thought Bobby would be dead," Bill Parcells said. "Yeah, almost every one of them. They said, 'Bill, that guy, he's headed fucking no place. He's done.'"

Parcells feels guilty he couldn't save Johnson from himself, even knowing from experience with other players that once they succumb to drugs, it's hard to get them back.

But then . . .

"Bobby walked in at the twenty-five-year reunion in 2011 with a cross around his neck," Parcells said.

He had to look twice to make sure it was him. They hugged, and Johnson assured him the "dark days" were over. "Shit, you're the last son of a bitch I expected to see," Parcells said.

"I've been sober for eleven years; I was homeless at times for fourteen years," Johnson said to his former coach.

Johnson didn't attend the ten-year anniversary in 1996. He was still using crack. Nobody knew where he was. "It was like Bobby was in the Witness Protection Program," Harry Carson said.

It was even more complicated than that.

"I mean, it's an unbelievable story," Parcells said.

———

BOBBY JOHNSON MADE the Giants as an undrafted free agent wide receiver from Kansas in 1984. He was born in Shelbyville, Tennessee, and came from a military family. His father was in the Air Force, and Bobby moved around a lot as a kid. His parents divorced when he was ten years old, and he lived with his mother, Ruby, in East St. Louis, one of the roughest areas in the country, until he went to play college football. After not getting drafted, he had several offers but picked the Giants over the Cowboys.

He smoked weed and drank in college, and when he arrived in New York, he didn't know anything about cocaine and had never even heard of crack. He liked women, he liked to drink, and he was part of Carl Banks's group of young players who would sleep in the Giants Stadium parking lot on Friday nights during the season, making the 9 a.m. team meeting after an evening of partying at Manhattan's finest clubs.

Johnson had an immediate impact on the Giants as a rookie, tying tight end Zeke Mowatt for the team lead with forty-eight catches and leading them with 795 yards receiving and seven touchdown catches. He started all sixteen regular season games. "Bobby was a great kid," wide receivers coach Pat Hodgson said. "Bobby had a great heart." The Giants finished 9–7 and earned a spot in the playoffs as a wild-card team. They beat the Rams in Anaheim in the first round but lost to the eventual Super Bowl champion 49ers in the divisional round.

"He was a good little player," Parcells said. "The son of a bitch could catch BBs in the dark. He really could. He wasn't real fast, but he had great hands and was quick out of his cuts."

Johnson was still starting in 1985, but second-year receiver Lionel Manuel led the Giants with forty-nine catches and 859 yards receiving despite playing three fewer games than Johnson. His catches dropped to thirty-three, and his yards went down to 533, but he led the Giants with eight touchdown receptions on an offense that relied on Joe Morris and the running game. The Giants once again made the playoffs as a wild-card team, beat the 49ers in the opening round, and lost in the divisional round once again to the team that would win the Super Bowl, this time the Bears.

Johnson was living in an apartment in Hackensack, just an easy fifteen-minute drive on Route 17 South to Giants Stadium. One of his friends was over at his apartment one night after practice during the middle of his second season, and they invited some women to join them. One of the female guests put cocaine on a table. The coke was arranged in lines, and for the first time in his life Johnson snorted. He liked it. A lot. Then somebody said, "Have you ever tried it like this?" One of the women had boiled cocaine with baking soda and water to produce white chunks that looked like small rocks. The woman put it in a pipe and Johnson smoked it. He found out it was called crack. He liked that even more.

"The rest is history," Johnson said. "It was the devil in disguise."

He loved the intense and quick high crack gave him. Loved the euphoric feeling. Felt invincible. His life was consumed with getting through practice and going out to find the next high. He was soon addicted. "I didn't know the symptoms. I didn't know what to look for," his mother, Ruby, said. "All I did was pray."

Lawrence Taylor was not in Johnson's apartment when he first experienced cocaine. Johnson won't say if he ever did crack with him, although it is fair to wonder. They had something in common. "Me and L.T. were probably the best friends of anybody on the team," Johnson said.

He insists Taylor was not a bad influence on him. He takes responsibility for his own drug habit. "Once you're addicted, ain't nobody influencing you to do that," he said. "That night when I done it, I was like, I'm not going to become addicted, you know. I didn't know crack was addictive because I didn't know what it was. I thought I had a strong enough will just to do it that night. You know, call it quits, never do it again."

The NFL in the '80s was not as diligent as it is today in recognizing a drug problem and getting a player the assistance he needs. Johnson said he would have welcomed the Giants sending him to a rehab center and regrets they didn't. But he never asked for help. He never thought about checking himself into rehab. Johnson was productive during the 1986 season despite his full-blown addiction. Teammates realized he was not as reliable off the field. He was late more than once reporting to the team plane for road games. "Parcells was so pissed off," Banks said. "It was a family situation, and Bobby was part of our family. We were pissed off at the player. You can't fucking do this. You can't be late. We were holding each other accountable."

The Giants were banged up at receiver, so Parcells had to keep playing Johnson. Simms trusted him to get open and catch the ball. And his catch against the Vikings led to the victory that convinced the Giants they could win the Super Bowl.

Before converting a first down on the play that became known simply as "Fourth and 17," Johnson's 25-yard touchdown catch with just under ten minutes left pushed the Giants in front of the Vikings 19–13. Minnesota came back to take the lead on Wade Wilson's 33-yard touchdown pass to Cris Carter halfway through the fourth quarter. Minnesota led 20–19, and after an exchange of punts, the Giants' three-game winning streak was in jeopardy as they started their drive at their own 41-yard line with 2:14 left. They were tied with Washington for first place in the NFC East and tied for the best record in the NFC. After losing on the road in the playoffs the previous two seasons, the Giants number-one goal in 1986 was to win the division and secure home field for the playoffs. Each game was crucial. The drive was crucial.

Johnson helped the Giants pick up a first down with a 14-yard catch over the middle. But after Ottis Anderson ran for two yards and Simms threw incomplete to Johnson, the Giants' quarterback was sacked for a 9-yard loss by Doug Martin, the younger brother of Giants defensive end George Martin. Parcells used the first of his three time-outs. The Giants were on their own 48. It was fourth down and a long 17 yards to go. Just 1:12 was left on the clock. They needed a big gain, if not a miracle, to keep the drive alive.

Down and distance were the enemy. The Giants had enough time and two timeouts remaining.

Simms came back to the huddle with the play:

Half Right W Motion 74 X In.

Simms still raves about Johnson's hands. Never drops the ball.

It was the first play the Giants installed in training camp in the summer, but the ball never went to Johnson when they practiced it. Simms told Johnson as they broke the huddle to be ready. Tight end Mark Bavaro was lined up 2 yards behind and to the right of right tackle Karl Nelson. But Bavaro whiffed trying to block Minnesota defensive tackle Keith Millard. As Simms was releasing the ball, Millard hit him. Johnson had run a perfect route between cornerback Issiac Holt and safety John Harris. Simms still had enough on the ball to drop it perfectly right between the two Vikings directly to Johnson along the right sideline. He tapped his toes to make sure he was in bounds before his momentum carried him out.

It was a 22-yard gain to the Vikings 30. The Giants were already in field goal range, but Parcells wanted to get closer for kicker Raul Allegre. A 5-yard encroachment penalty on Martin and runs of 8, 2, and 0 yards by Morris moved the Giants to the Vikings 15-yard line and positioned New York for Allegre's 33-yard field goal attempt. His kick went through with twelve seconds remaining, and the Giants had a hard-earned 22–20 victory.

"Had it not been for that combination of Simms to Bobby Johnson, I might not be wearing a Super Bowl ring," Carson said.

"We did get on a freaking roll," Johnson said. "We got the feeling after that game that we were unbeatable. We didn't lose a game after that."

"After that Bobby Johnson catch, nobody played with us," Taylor said.

Johnson did not make a spectacular catch. It was routine and at any other point in the game would not have been memorable. But he did everything right at the most important time. He ran a great route, made sure there was enough room between his feet and the boundary, brought the ball in with both hands, and stepped out. His catch along with Bavaro's catch and run against the 49ers two weeks later are the two signature plays on the road to the Super Bowl.

"To me, it was just a normal play," Johnson said. "And it was an easy catch."

On the twenty-year anniversary of the 1986 Giants Super Bowl season, I visited Johnson at his mother's home in Smyrna, Tennessee. By then, he had been off cocaine for about five years and was working hard to get his life straightened out. He was living on the streets and then not living on the streets. That went on for too long. Ruby took him in occasionally. I brought a DVD of the documentary produced by NFL Films of the Giants Super Bowl season so we could view the fourth-and-17 play together. As Johnson intently watched himself make the catch, he cried and turned off the DVD player in his mother's living room. It was bittersweet. He knows he could have had a great career, and "Fourth and 17" is a reminder of how good he was, how much Simms trusted him, and how much he screwed up what could have been a long, lucrative career. He said he could only watch that play again by himself. I left the DVD with him.

"I get as emotional as he does," Ruby said. "It just seems that was another life."

The Giants finished off the season by winning the NFC East, earning a first-round bye and home field in the conference playoffs. Johnson's numbers once again took a tumble. He led the Giants wide receivers but with only thirty-one catches for 534 yards and five touchdowns even as injuries limited Manuel and Stacy Robinson. In the divisional round, when the Giants demolished San Francisco 49–3, Johnson had only one catch for 15 yards, and it was for a touchdown. Simms attempted just nineteen passes, completing nine, as the Giants gashed the 49ers on the ground for 216 yards on forty-four carries.

One more victory, and they would be in their first Super Bowl.

The atmosphere in New York leading up to the NFC Championship Game against Washington was festive. It had been thirty years since the Giants had won their last championship. Even the rival Jets, who came into the AFL as the Titans in 1960, had won a Super Bowl. The Giants defeated Washington twice during the regular season, including the division-deciding game on the road in early December, and as difficult as it's supposed to be to beat a team—especially a very good team—three times in one season, the Giants were confident they were going to beat Washington. Johnson was feeling good about himself as a player after catching the touchdown against the 49ers despite turning into a crackhead off the field.

As usual, the Giants had meetings and a walk-through on Saturday morning, the day before the game. They had the afternoon off and then checked into their hotel in Woodcliff Lake, far enough from Manhattan that only players looking to blow curfew would take a chance crossing the river and making it back in time.

Kickoff for the NFC Championship game was just after 4 p.m., following the AFC title game between the Broncos and Browns in Cleveland, which was kicking off at 12:30 p.m. Even with the later start time, no player could possibly be so selfish, immature, and stupid to risk costing his team a shot at the Super Bowl by showing up late for the game. No player who cared about his teammates would sneak out of the hotel in the middle of the night after curfew in pursuit of sex or drugs.

Except Bobby Johnson.

PARCELLS SET AN 11 p.m. curfew, the same as it had been all season. The players were on their own the next morning until reporting to the stadium two to three hours before the game. The coach was aware that two or three of his players would always sneak out after bed check and curfew, but they were adults so he wanted to trust them. If he caught them, they would be fined. But it was not as if Parcells was sitting in the hotel lobby that night and stationed his assistants by the side entrances to monitor his players. If they were willing to risk hurting the team this close to the Super Bowl, it would show up on the field and eventually cost them their job.

That didn't enter Johnson's mind when a female friend invited him over to her place to smoke crack. It was 3 a.m.—he said it might even have been as late as 4 a.m.—when he sneaked out of his hotel room in North Jersey, got in his car, and drove forty-five miles all the way to Rockaway Beach on the southern edge of Queens not far from Kennedy Airport. That meant crossing virtually all of New York City, including multiple bridges. At that time of the night, it takes a little more than an hour. But on Sunday, he knew the return trip would be longer—perhaps much longer. He would need to get an early start to make it to the stadium by 2 p.m. at the latest. Regardless of whether he worked his way back to New Jersey through Brooklyn on the Belt Parkway to the Verrazzano Bridge and through Staten Island or took the Whitestone Bridge to the Bronx and hopped on the dreaded Cross Bronx Expressway to the George Washington Bridge, he was going to encounter massive traffic. Longtime Giants fans from New York use those routes and have complained since the team moved to Jersey in 1976 about the maddening game-day traffic jams. The aggravating drive convinced many of them to cancel their season tickets and watch on television at home.

Johnson naturally made it far worse for himself by oversleeping after bingeing on crack. He looked at his watch when he woke up. It was 2:15 p.m. Kickoff was at 4:04 p.m. "The first thing I thought of was I just fucked up and I was letting the team down," Johnson said. "I knew I would also feel the wrath of Coach Parcells."

Now the race was on to get to East Rutherford in time for kick-off and pray Parcells would let him play. He didn't get in his car until 2:45 p.m. The most important game of his life was starting in seventy-nine minutes, and he not only was already late but he was nowhere near Giants Stadium.

He did not win the race by much. When the traffic slowed down before he even neared the stadium, Johnson flagged down a New Jersey state trooper and begged for an escort. "I'm late for the game, sir," he told the trooper. "Please give me help as far as you can go."

When the traffic soon came to a dead stop, the escort was over, and Johnson was on his own the rest of the way. By the time he arrived in the locker room, the Giants were back in from the pregame warm-ups, and kickoff was in fifteen minutes. He had royally screwed up. His absence didn't go unnoticed by his teammates and coaches. When they didn't see him in warm-ups, they knew there was trouble. It was not the first time they questioned his commitment to the team. But this was the worst.

"Well, first of all, we go out for warm-ups, he's not there," Parcells said. "We come back in, he's not there. Everybody knows he is not there."

Johnson sprinted down the ramp from the players' parking lot, rushed into the locker room, and was immediately confronted by Taylor and Jim Burt. It was not a pleasant encounter. They wanted to beat the shit out of him. Even with all his drug problems, Taylor's teammates knew they never had to worry about him getting to the stadium on time or being the best player on the field for sixty minutes. Johnson didn't have that benefit of the doubt.

If this was a regular-season game, Parcells would have benched Johnson and likely cut him the next day. But the Giants were playing to get into the Super Bowl, and he was concerned about his depth at wide receiver if he ordered Johnson to take off his uniform. Without him, the Giants would have only four receivers: Manuel, Robinson, Phil McConkey, and Solomon Miller. Any injury in the game would be crippling, forcing the offensive coaches to cut plays out of their game plan and thrusting players into unfamiliar roles. Parcells was also not aware Johnson had snuck out of the hotel, driven to Queens, and done crack all night. "I knew something was wrong, but I was not sure what it was," Parcells said.

Simms was obviously aware Johnson was not taking his place in the receiver line in the warm-ups but was too focused on the game to worry about it. As the Giants paraded off the field following the pre-game activities, Simms saw Johnson running down the ramp. "I had no idea what was happening," he said. Parcells was in the coaches locker room going over last-minute details with his staff when two of his defensive players frantically charged in to get him.

"Jerome Sally and John Washington come running back and go, 'Bill, Bill. They're killing him. They're killing him.' So, I go out and there he is, they got Bobby down in the middle of the floor. I mean, you know, Taylor, Burt, their lockers were right there when he walks through the door. They pounced on him like panthers," Parcells said. "They got him down. Burt gets him up. He rips his fucking clothes off. They run him down to the locker and say, 'You better fucking play, you little motherfucker.' There's like eight or ten of them. This is going on while I'm en route to get into this mess. But they're saying, 'You better play, you little motherfucker. You won't leave here alive today.' They are threatening the son of a bitch."

Burt laughs recalling the confrontation. He remembers he and Taylor scared the hell out of Johnson, but he said they didn't have a chance to get physical with him because Johnson ran away from them. Taylor's drug problems were an unspoken truth, but the depth of Johnson's issues were not necessarily common knowledge in the locker room. Burt didn't know why Johnson was late and didn't care. "We chased him into the training room. We chased him not really wanting to catch him," he said. "Basically, it was to show the other guys how serious we were and how big a game this was. If Bobby didn't run a little faster, yes, he would've got it."

Johnson sheepishly said, "Nobody touched me or anything like that. It was just, 'Where you been? You know how important this is.' They got in my face."

He quickly put on his uniform No. 88 and ran out with the team for introductions and the national anthem. "There's a few guys on each team who you really like but they are fuckups. Bobby was one of those guys," Burt said. "Being late for the game was totally irresponsible and way over the line."

It was contrary to everything the disciplined Parcells believed in to allow Johnson to play. If the media had known about it at the time, Parcells would have been criticized for not sending Johnson home. He not only played but started. Nearly forty years later, Parcells offered no regrets letting Johnson play. "He got there in time for the game," he said.

Parcells insists he was actually putting the team first by dealing with Johnson later. "We would have been short receivers if I benched him," he said. "You can't do that to your team. You can't punish everybody else."

Johnson did not have a catch against Washington. Simms threw only fourteen passes and completed seven in the swirling winds of Giants Stadium. Two weeks later in the Super Bowl, Johnson again started and did not catch a pass. He thinks Parcells told Simms to freeze him out because "I wasn't getting no balls in practice, let alone the game. That touchdown catch against the 49ers was the last pass I ever caught. In the Washington game, I didn't even have a pass thrown my way."

Parcells wouldn't have played Johnson at all before telling Simms not to throw him the ball. He wasn't good enough to just be a decoy, and the Giants in effect would have been playing 10-on-11. But Johnson's tardiness was his eventual ticket out of town.

Once they made it past Washington, Parcells put a plan in place to prevent Johnson from creating any kind of a distraction when the Giants arrived in Southern California for the Super Bowl one week before the game. There were just too many temptations. Parcells was friends with a retired NFL player who didn't play for the Giants and paid him a few hundred dollars for the week to keep an eye on Johnson around the clock.

"I ain't going to fuck up this game." Parcells said. "You stay with this son of a bitch. I want to know anything he does."

He didn't put a tail on Taylor. Johnson, in his mind, was much more liable to get himself into trouble. Parcells had the former player he hired check in with him constantly. The first day he came back with some potentially bad news.

"Coach, he wrote a check for $2,500," he said.

Parcells had no doubt where the money went. "So, I'm saying to myself, he's buying dope, you know?" he said. He summoned Johnson to his office. Parcells knew Johnson was scared of him and he went into attack mode.

"I see you wrote a check for $2,500. What did you do?" Parcells said.

"I bought a camcorder to record Super Bowl week," Johnson said.

Parcells was skeptical.

"Go get the receipt," he said.

Johnson went up to his hotel room and came down with a receipt for $1,700.

"Where's the other $800?" Parcells demanded.

Johnson took out the cash.

"Here's $100 for the day," Parcells said.

Parcells gave the other $700 to the former player. Johnson's teammates punished him for showing up late for the championship game by making him the official team videographer for the week.

Johnson knew his time with the Giants was coming to an end by the time he made it to training camp in 1987. New York had taken three wide receivers early in the draft: Mark Ingram in the first round, Stephen Baker in the third round, and Odessa Turner in the fourth. Parcells was well aware Johnson had a cocaine problem, and since his value was considerably less than Taylor's, he didn't have the same patience with him, as much as he liked him as a player.

"I traded him after the season," Parcells said. "You know what was sad about him was that I really liked him. He just got off track and didn't come back for a long time. At the reunion, he gives me a hug and says, 'You saved my life.' I like him. All the players liked him. The little son of a bitch was a good competitor now. If he was out there, you could count on him. He had good hands. He was quick. I mean, he was just a fuckup."

Parcells sent Johnson to the San Diego Chargers during camp. He lasted three weeks and was cut seven days before the start of the season. He never played in the NFL again. His last game was the Super Bowl victory. He cried to running back Tony Galbreath on the bench as the Giants started to celebrate in the final minutes. He knew Parcells was going to get rid of him. He authored his own demise.

"That one night changed my whole life as far as my football career," Johnson said. "Parcells said I was doing good and people liked me, but you came to that game late and you can't do that. When they traded me, they said my urine had cocaine in it. I had nothing in my system. I knew I was going to get tested at the beginning of camp in July and came into the season after the Super Bowl clean as hell. Cocaine only stays in your system three days. I was clean, but I was still getting punished for coming to that game late. Even though I was clean, who knows if I would have relapsed the second or third game of the season. They did the right thing."

No NFL. No more drug tests. He could smoke all the crack he could afford. And he did day and night.

"I started right back," he said.

Even players who don't have a drug problem are often lost after football. They've never considered what the rest of their life will look like. A fortunate few get a job in broadcast media, actually took college seriously and make productive use of their degree, go back to school to complete their degree, or go into the family business. Johnson did none of that. He had no family business. His father was in the military. Johnson had no plans for a second career, had a serious drug problem, and soon ran out of money. Football was over for him four months before his twenty-sixth birthday. What was next? He had to figure that out much earlier than anticipated.

"Life wasn't the same without football," he said. "It was a culture shock. I didn't know what else to do. It was the only thing I wanted to do all my life. I just started to get down on myself. I actually went into a deep depression."

No team was touching a player with drug issues unless he was a superstar. Johnson moved back to Nashville, and his mother was living nearby in Smyrna. Johnson had a young son from a college relationship he didn't see from the age of four until twenty years later when he got cleaned up. He knew his drug use was destroying his mother. She had to throw him out of her apartment several times to preserve her sanity.

"Your mama is always going to take you in," Johnson said. "I could have knocked on her door some night, but she would have eventually thrown me out again. She wanted me to be clean. She said don't come back until you are clean or until you try and start. I couldn't see my family. Truly, nobody wanted me around. I don't blame them. To this day, I apologize. I got clean when I just got fed up."

For fifteen years, beginning after he was cut in 1987, Johnson's addiction consumed every dollar and thought he had. His life became a somber movie. He worked day laborer jobs, some for $10 an hour, others that paid him $150–$200 in a day, and he spent it on drugs. He was completely homeless for one year. In the evenings, he would lie down on a bench in Riverfront Park on Second Avenue in downtown Nashville next to the site that later became the Tennessee Titans stadium. If concerts were not going on, the area was dangerous after dark. He never closed his eyes, counting the minutes until the sun would come up. In the winter, he would shiver on the park bench, praying he would not freeze to death. One night he was praying he wouldn't take a bullet to his back. "Somebody wanted my drugs," he said. "He shot at me while I was running away. Thank God he couldn't shoot straight."

During the darkest days of his crack addiction, Johnson was arrested for possession of marijuana and writing a bad check.

He had mental health issues. He had financial issues. Then, he had a physical issue.

Johnson had a job at a pencil manufacturing plant in 1994 in the Nashville suburb of Shelbyville where he was born. And there he suffered an injury far worse than anything that happened to him on the field.

"Another crushing moment in my life," he said.

He had been working at the industrial plant for a couple of years. He was wearing a pair of gloves, and the machine he was assigned to had two flat rollers side by side. "My glove caught in there and pulled my hand down," he said. "I had to yank it out. It was four hundred degrees."

He lost the three fingers down to the second knuckle and needed skin grafts to replace the skin on the back of his hand. The skin is so dark compared to the rest of his hand that it looks like he's wearing a glove.

He found parts of his middle, ring, and pinkie fingers of his right hand lying on the other side of the rollers. Blood was splattered everywhere. "It didn't cut them off. It pulled them off," he said. "I had to pull my arm back out because my body was going in, too."

Sitting with his mother as he told this part of his story in 2007, Johnson grabbed a piece of paper off the coffee table. "My fingers were as flat as this paper," he said. "I call them three popsicle sticks."

The plant closed one week after the accident. Johnson never collected one penny in compensation for what happened to him.

Johnson would sometimes sleep in a shelter if he arrived in time to get a bed. He was so desperate for money he stole checks from his mother. "The drug dealers actually knew me, so they would give me stuff on credit," he said in 2022. "I would give them my Super Bowl ring sometimes, get a job, pay them back and get the ring back. Yeah, it was a revolving door. I don't want nobody to live like that. Nobody wants to be addicted and homeless. It's double ridiculous. You get lonely and it's dangerous. It's dangerous down there. They try to take your drugs, your food, and your clothes. I finally just got tired. I had to just get on my knees and start praying, 'Lord, I don't want to do this no more.' At the time you're thinking you are going to be addicted all your life. This is how it's going to be the rest of your life. Eventually you just got to say no."

Before he could finally say no, "you get crazy thoughts," he said.

Johnson's painful journey led him on an exceedingly cold night from the park bench to what was then known as the Shelby Street Bridge, a pedestrian bridge over the Cumberland River that connects downtown Nashville with a residential area in East Nashville. It is one of the longest pedestrian bridges in the world, at 3,150 feet.

The river almost became the burial ground for Bobby Johnson in 2002.

Suicidal thoughts had been running through his mind for some time. He hated what he had become. "I didn't want to live like that for the rest of my life," he said.

He walked on the bridge. He positioned one of his legs over the railing. This was a homeless man, a former football star, who had come under the thrall of addiction. He was a long way from "Fourth and 17" hanging thirty-nine feet above the Cumberland River.

"When I was sitting up on that bridge that night, I didn't have no money, no nothing, just wanting to get high. Oh my God, sitting on top of that bridge," he said as his voice trails off.

Johnson couldn't bring himself to lift his other leg over the railing and jump. He was maybe more scared of heights than he was of dying. He was ready to jump into the freezing water and give up on his life, but the thirty-nine feet looked as high up as the top of the Empire State Building as Johnson straddled the railing. "I don't like heights," he said. "That's what got me down off the bridge, actually. I literally said to myself, 'You stupid ass. You're afraid of heights anyway. Get your dumb ass down and get your life together.'"

"It was cold as shit, too."

He was so addicted to cocaine that not even the close call with death convinced him to never smoke crack again. "I relapsed probably fifty times after that night, you know what I'm saying?" he said.

Johnson eventually scared himself straight. The date will stick in his mind forever.

"December 3, 2002," he said.

It was the end of an eventful year.

＝＝＝

JOHNSON LOCKED HIMSELF in his mother's apartment until he felt secure that he would not be tempted to do drugs or have any contact with drug dealers. He didn't attempt to get a job during that time. He was completely focused on finding a way to stop breaking his mother's heart and setting himself up with a productive life. He could only guess how things might have turned out with the Giants if drugs hadn't sabotaged his career. There was money to be made for being Bobby Johnson, Super Bowl champion.

Considering where he was, it's not so bad where he is now. He reconnected with his son. He bought a house with his girlfriend Brenda, who he's been with since 2010, in Murfreesboro, Tennessee, a three-hour drive from his mother. After settling down by working eight years for NHK, a company that makes seats for Nissan cars, he's now a warehouse operation lead at NFI Distribution Center in Smyrna. He's reconnected with Giants teammates and is a regular at reunion events. He's happy around the Super Bowl group, and they are happy he is back. "I'm living my best life," he said.

There was one bit of unfinished business as Johnson was checking off boxes to put his troubles behind him. He desperately wanted the Super Bowl XXI ring he'd pawned. He hocked it for $450 even though he was offered $1,000. He intentionally kept the amount low, figuring it would be easier to come up with the funds to pay it back. He walked into the Rose Loan Company at 419 Broadway in Nashville on September 23, 1989, and signed a contract labeled "Pawn #14775." When he failed to pay back the money in the fifty days plus ten days' grace period outlined in the contract, the diamond ring with Johnson's name inscribed no longer belonged to him.

Alan Joseph, a lawyer who lived at the time in Plainview, Long Island, was well known to the players as a big-time Giants collector. He was born in 1940 and was a second cousin of Giants radio broadcaster

Marty Glickman, who used to help him get tickets to games. Joseph owns 256 plaques with Giants helmets and pictures signed by the players. He has a collection of 150,000 Giants trading cards. His old office in Glendale, Queens, was twenty feet by one hundred feet, and every inch of the wall was taken up by Giants memorabilia. He has been to each of the Giants five Super Bowl games.

He also attended Super Bowl XXXIV in Atlanta between the St. Louis Rams and Tennessee Titans on January 30, 2000. In the days before the game, he went to the NFL Experience, and one of the shops was selling football collector items.

"His name was the Ring Man," Joseph said.

Joseph was immediately attracted to one ring: Bobby Johnson's Super Bowl XXI ring. The Ring Man purchased it from the pawn shop. Joseph had become friends with many of the Giants from the '86 team and contacted George Martin to get his opinion whether the ring was real. The Ring Man provided authentication papers.

The price: $10,000.

Sold to the lawyer from New York.

Joseph now had Bobby Johnson's Super Bowl XXI ring to add to his collection. He had become friends with Giants wide receiver Stacy Robinson, who knew Joseph was trying to find Johnson to let him know he had the ring. Robinson was on business in the Midwest in his role with the NFL Players Association when he made the acquaintance of a drug counselor from Tennessee who coincidentally had come in contact with Johnson. Robinson, through the drug counselor, hooked up Johnson and Joseph. They became friendly. At one of the Giants reunions with Johnson still battling hard times, Joseph loaned him $1,500, which Johnson never repaid. On another visit, Johnson spent the day with Joseph at his house.

On one of his trips to New York, Joseph handed Johnson the ring and let him wear it. "That was torture," Johnson told me in 2007. "I didn't want to take it off. If I get it back, I think that would turn my life around. That's a crazy thing to say, but certain things in life do that to you."

It was a tease to see the ring and a bigger one to wear it. It seemed like the end of the world to give it back.

In the joyous locker room after the Super Bowl, Parcells stood in front of his team and told them, "The rest of your life, men, nobody can tell you that you couldn't do it, because you did it."

The words were all Johnson had left from the championship. He had nothing tangible to show for his Giants career. While Johnson's teammates had become attorneys or financial planners or entrepreneurs or tried to make a living just being Lawrence Taylor, he had put himself through hell and finally come out the other side. But knowing he didn't have his ring, or any real possession linked to his Super Bowl championship, gnawed at him. It could feel like the memory wasn't quite real.

As Johnson was feeling better about himself, he began to speak to patients at drug rehabilitation centers, telling his cautionary story. He was an aberration. He willed himself to get clean on his own without even checking into rehab himself. When he finally decided to stop using drugs, he showed the same mental toughness he displayed going over the middle knowing he was about to get drilled by a safety or linebacker. He brought the story I wrote about him in the *New York Daily News* on the twenty-year anniversary of the Super Bowl to rehab centers to hang on the wall.

But still—it didn't mean quite the same thing without the ring.

The Super Bowl XXI rings were distributed by the Giants to players, coaches, and staff before the 1987 season. By 1989, Johnson's was in a pawn shop.

Nine years after Johnson told the story of the pawned ring to me, he told it to Michelle Beisner-Buck in an ESPN feature on *Monday Night Countdown* before the Giants played the Vikings on October 3, 2016. It was thirty years earlier in the old Metrodome in downtown Minneapolis, on the same site as the new US Bank Stadium, where Johnson made his most significant contribution to the Super Bowl season.

New York businessman Lee Einsidler, a big Giants fan and CEO of Casamigos Tequila, saw the ESPN feature and was touched by Johnson's story. He was good friends with Parcells and Wellington Mara's son Chris, a Giants vice president. Parcells, Mara, and Einsidler share a love of horse racing, and all own a few thoroughbreds. (Mara owns a share of 2018 Triple Crown winner Justify and 2020 Kentucky Derby winner Authentic.)

It was Einsidler who provided the impetus to help Johnson.

"He comes to us and says, 'We need to get this fucking guy's ring back,'" Parcells said.

Parcells first wanted to be reassured Johnson had remained clean since he last spoke with him at the 2011 reunion of the '86 team. Parcells was very encouraged at the time, but another five years had passed. A lot of bad things for a recovering addict could happen in a day, no less five years. After doing his research, Parcells was satisfied Johnson had not relapsed and got on board in the search for the ring.

"I think he's out of the woods," Parcells said. "I think he's doing okay. I would know if he wasn't."

Parcells called Johnson to check up on him and told him he was going to try to do something for him. Johnson told him he knew who had the ring and gave him Joseph's phone number. Johnson was at work when he spoke to Parcells and was so excited he couldn't function and had to leave early.

"We finally were able to run it down," Parcells said. "After that, we just did what we had to do."

By then, Joseph had moved to a townhouse in Melville, Long Island. The property manager was Einsidler's brother. "Everybody knew I had the ring," Joseph said. He told Joseph that his brother Lee wanted to buy the ring. Lee called to set up an appointment to meet in Joseph's office and informed him he was a good friend of Parcells. "I really didn't want to sell it except that it was going back to Bobby," Joseph said. "Otherwise, I absolutely was not going to part with it."

Joseph and Einsidler negotiated. Joseph wanted more than Einsidler wanted to pay. Einsidler offered less than Joseph wanted. They compromised.

The price was $30,000. In less than one week, Einsidler was in Joseph's office with a certified check for $30,000.

Parcells said he paid $15,000 and Einsidler paid $15,000.

It took them less than two weeks to find the ring, pay for it, and present it to Johnson. On October 16, 2016, the Giants hosted seventy former players on their annual alumni weekend for a game against the Baltimore Ravens. During a pregame event, Joann Lamneck, the Giants alumni and community relations manager, pulled Johnson aside and told him he was wanted in a private area of the stadium. Johnson had been conditioned to expect the worst: What did I do wrong?

Chris Mara was standing by himself with a ring box in his left hand as Johnson walked toward him. When he reached Mara, the two men hugged. "So, thirty years ago, my dad presented you with your Super Bowl ring," Mara said. "Through the efforts of some very good people, Bill Parcells, your old coach, my good friend Lee Einsidler, and myself, we were able to recover your ring after all these years. We want to present it to you today."

Mara opened the box and handed it to Johnson. He immediately put the ring on his finger.

"Oh my God, oh my God," Johnson said. "Thank you very much."

He hugged Mara again. Then he cried. He walked a few feet to sit down and sobbed uncontrollably with his head in his hands. Mara sat next to him rubbing his back. After a few minutes, Mara called Parcells and put Johnson on the phone. Parcells told him to put the ring on and never take it off. Parcells, the tough guy coach, has developed a paternal feeling toward his former players, even the ones who messed up. He believed Johnson was a big part of the '86 Giants, was off drugs, and deserved the ring.

"It was great," Parcells said in an interview posted on the Giants team website. "What's nice is that I must have had fifteen texts from all the other players that were there. They were all thanking me. It makes you feel good. That's what a team is supposed to be. They're supposed to care about each other. That team, that's what that team did and still does. That's great."

Johnson still is perplexed and distraught about how he could go from a success as an undrafted rookie free agent to drug addict to Super Bowl champion to homeless. What's most important to him now is his girlfriend, his son, and his mother. And staying clean and keeping his job. He was one of seven hundred former players who benefited from a change in the 2020 collective bargaining agreement that reduced the vested period from three seasons plus three games down to three seasons. "I qualify," Johnson said. His pension pays $19,800 annually for life.

He came to New York for the Giants 2022 reunion. He didn't hide his right hand and showed off his left, which had a beautiful Super Bowl diamond ring he wears as often as possible. It was the rare case of Cinderella getting back her glass slipper. "I love life," he said.

Three words he never thought he would say again.

Johnson is back in the Giants family. There is no place he would rather be.

8

FAMILY VALUES

NFL commissioner Pete Rozelle held the Vince Lombardi Trophy in his right hand as he stood on a podium set up in the noisy and cramped Giants locker room in the Rose Bowl. Wellington Mara was to his immediate left, and CBS broadcaster Brent Musburger and Bill Parcells were to his far left. It had been thirty years since the Giants won a championship, and the years in between had mostly been miserable.

John Mara, the oldest of the eleven Mara children, was thirty-two years old at Super Bowl XXI and not yet working for the team. He was an attorney in Manhattan specializing in labor and employment law and litigation. He lived and died with every Giants game and was emotional, unlike his stoic father. He's been known to throw or kick things when a game is going poorly. John once lost his job as a spotter for CBS football broadcasts after working "The Fumble" game in 1978. He slammed his fist on a table, sending all kinds of electronic equipment flying, as he watched Herm Edwards scoop up the loose ball and run untouched for the winning touchdown. Years later, as co-owner of the team, he's been known to toss a trash can or two in his suite at MetLife Stadium. He no longer sits in the press box at Giants road games, a tradition started by his father, and instead retreats to the owner's suite so potential outbursts are kept under wraps.

He endured his father being heavily and at times viciously criticized for the Giants' ineptitude, the worst coming in the weeks after Joe Pisarcik's infamous fumble, when fans burned tickets in a portable toilet bowl in the Giants Stadium parking lot and the next week rented an airplane to fly over the stadium during a game with a banner that read, *"15 Yrs of Lousy Football. We've Had Enough."* That prompted Andy Robustelli, an all-time Giants great who was the team's director of football operations, to comment, "I was a 20-millimeter gunner in the service. I wish I had it then and I would have blown the plane right out of the sky."

John Mara was standing just a few feet from the podium watching his father embrace the Super Bowl XXI trophy moments after the 39–20 victory over the Denver Broncos. His view was spectacular, the greatest sight he could ever imagine, on a stage seemingly reserved for Art Rooney of the Steelers, Tex Schramm of the Cowboys, Joe Robbie of the Dolphins, and Lombardi himself.

"After a long spell of not having very good teams, the fan protests and all that stuff, to finally win a Super Bowl, to finally see my father on the platform in the locker room in Pasadena accepting the Lombardi Trophy, was very special for my family," John Mara reflected more than thirty-five years later.

Wellington Mara said a few words, praising his players and coaches, and handed the trophy to Parcells. When CBS came back from commercial, Rozelle was gone and Mara and Parcells had been replaced by Tim Mara, whose side of the family owned 50 percent of the Giants, and George Young, the general manager. It was no accident Wellington and Tim didn't appear together and no accident Parcells and Young were kept separate. Parcells had no use for Young after he plotted to replace him following his first season as head coach in 1983. The hatred between the two Maras ran even deeper, and if fans were not aware or had forgotten about the "War of the Roses," dysfunction in the family that had been publicly—but not privately—dormant since Young was hired in 1979, it was about to go national.

First, Young said, "I'm happy for both sides of the Mara family . . ."

That was the first clue that this was not one big happy Mara family.

Then Musburger let it rip with Young to his left and Tim Mara to his right: "George and Tim, I don't want to sensationalize the point, nor do I want to leave without referring to it. That's the fact that Wellington and Tim do not get along. But the fact remains they kept the focus on winning football games, they got the job done this year, and they deserve to be acclaimed for that."

Not since Rozelle was forced to hand the Lombardi Trophy to his archenemy Al Davis of the Raiders had there been such drama on the podium. It was as a result of the Mara family feud that the NFL eventually implemented a rule to require each team that was sold to designate a partner with controlling interest if no one person held 51 percent. If the rule had been instituted earlier, it could have saved the Giants aggravation and humiliation.

Wellington's father, Tim, was a legal bookmaker. He had an opportunity in 1925 to invest $500 in the career of heavyweight boxer Gene Tunney but instead took the $500 to pay the entry fee to buy his way into the NFL with the New York Football Giants. The league started play in 1920 and became known as the National Football League in 1922. As a way to protect the Giants from creditors after the stock market crash in 1929, Tim split up ownership of the team in 1930. His older son Jack received 50 percent. His younger son Wellington received 50 percent. Jack was twenty-two. Wellington was fourteen. Tim continued to run the Giants until 1946, when he placed Wellington in charge of the football operation and Jack in charge of the business side.

Tim died in 1959 at the age of seventy-one. He was voted into the first class of the Pro Football Hall of Fame in 1963. The 50 percent he left to each of his sons was no longer simply for paperwork purposes. It was real. His death didn't change how the Giants functioned right away, but trouble loomed down the road. Wellington and Jack worked well together, and the Giants were successful on the field. Everything changed when Jack lost his battle with cancer in 1965. He was fifty-seven years old. His 50 percent went to his wife Helen, daughter Maura, and son Tim, who was designated to handle their share. Tim had been around the team most of his adult life, and franchise icon Frank Gifford once said Tim was his closest friend during his rookie season in 1952.

It didn't take long for things to go sideways after Jack died. Wellington was nineteen years older than his nephew. He was a religious family man with eleven children. Tim was divorced and very much enjoyed the New York nightlife. Wellington and Tim were from different generations with little in common. Wellington was still running the football side, Tim in time took over the business affairs as vice president and treasurer, but as the team was missing the playoffs year after year, Tim felt the need to speak up and protect his family's share. The Giants had been to six of the eight NFL championship games from 1956 to 1963, and although they lost the prior five, including the '58 overtime game to the Colts that's been called the greatest game ever played, they had big-name celebrity fan favorites Charlie Conerly, Y. A. Tittle, Gifford, and Sam Huff.

In the late '50s, Lombardi was the team's offensive coordinator, and Tom Landry was its defensive coordinator. Lombardi was hired to coach the Packers in 1959, and Landry, who intended to move back to his native Texas and go into private business, was hired to coach the expansion Cowboys in 1960 after nearly taking a job as head coach of the Houston Oilers of the new AFL. Wellington Mara recommended Landry to Schramm, who was the Cowboys president and general manager. Landry and Mara were close friends, and after Landry left New York to coach the Cowboys, they would have dinner with their wives each year before the Giants played in Dallas. Either Lombardi or Landry, future Hall of Famers, would have been the perfect replacement for Jim Lee Howell, but he didn't retire until after the 1960 season. The Giants tried and failed to get Lombardi to return, but even though he was from Sheepshead Bay in Brooklyn and later coached and taught at a New Jersey high school, he was reluctant to leave Green Bay after just two seasons. If he had come back and won the first two Super Bowls for the Giants instead of the Packers, Lombardi certainly would have been celebrated with more than a rest stop named after him on the New Jersey Turnpike.

With Howell retired and Lombardi in Green Bay and Landry in Dallas, the Giants were stuck. They promoted Allie Sherman, who in his second stint as an assistant with the team took over for Lombardi as offensive coordinator. Sherman lost in the NFL Championship Game his first three seasons as head coach. By his fourth year, he decided the Giants needed to be rebuilt and traded the very popular Huff to Washington. Huff never forgave Sherman. The Giants went from the championship game in 1963 to 2–10–2 in 1964. During a 1966 game at D.C. Stadium, Huff was screaming at Sherman on the opposite sideline and implored Washington coach Otto Graham to run up the score. The Giants lost 72–41.

The '64 season began a stretch of seventeen consecutive seasons in which the Giants failed to make the playoffs. Chants of "Goodbye Allie" reverberated through Yankee Stadium. Disgruntled fans took the chant across the border when the Giants played a preseason game in Montreal in 1969. "Goodbye Allie" was chanted in French. Earlier in the summer, the Giants were crushed by the Super Bowl champion Jets in their first-ever meeting in a preseason game at the Yale Bowl. Wellington Mara had seen enough and fired Sherman after a 0–5 preseason one week before the start of the regular season and replaced him by promoting former Giants running back Alex Webster.

Webster became a symbol of how Mara set the franchise back by rewarding former players with key positions when they were not the most qualified. Webster was a great Giants player; he was not a great Giants coach. He was 29–40–1 in five seasons before resigning. Too loyal in a league that only rewards loyalty if it results in victories, Mara held on to veteran scouts too long. He was still very involved in personnel decisions. The league was evolving, but the Giants were not. As the Cowboys took a step to the future introducing computers to scouting, the Giants were stuck in the '50s. In what was seen by the league at the time as an attempt to modernize the organization, the Giants hired cheerleaders in the early '70s. During pregame introductions, the cheerleaders made their first mistake: holding up cards to cheer on the team:

OG GIANTS OG

The transposing of letters was comical.

The cheerleaders were fired after the game, and the team has never rehired cheerleaders.

Pisarcik's 1978 play, called in the huddle as "Pro 65 UP," but later known to everyone simply as "The Fumble," was the low point in Giants history. But it was also an agent for much-needed change. Coach John McVay was fired after the '78 season. Robustelli, who had been hired by Wellington Mara in 1974, had told Mara before the 1978 season he would be leaving to run his travel agency after the season. Mara attempted to talk him out of it in midseason, around the time the Giants were 5–3 with a chance to end their playoff drought, but Tim Mara wrote a letter to Robustelli, informing him his decision was irrevocable. The Giants finished 6–10 by losing seven of their last eight games.

The Giants were a family-run business. Football was their only business. The business was suffering.

By the end of the season, Tim believed his uncle had run the team into the ground. Tim was no longer content sticking to the business side when the football side was hurting the business. He was determined to have input in the search for new leadership.

It turned into a public embarrassment.

The Giants needed a new football decision maker and a head coach and staff. Wellington wanted to promote Terry Bledsoe, whom he'd hired one year earlier as Robustelli's assistant without Tim Mara's knowledge. Tim vetoed Bledsoe moving up. The Giants went after Penn State coach Joe Paterno. He said no. Tim wanted George Allen, the former coach of Washington and the Rams. Wellington did not. Wellington interviewed Cowboys assistant Dan Reeves without telling Tim. When Tim called Reeves to ask him about it, he denied talking to

Wellington, but Reeves then had Landry call Tim to apologize for lying to him, saying Wellington had sworn him to secrecy.

The Maras asked Rozelle to get involved. Wellington and Tim couldn't agree on a new general manager (they did agree to update the title from director of football operations). They couldn't agree on a coach. They couldn't agree which of the two positions to hire first. (Most teams go with a GM and let him pick the coach.) Rozelle asked Wellington and Tim to list their top four candidates for GM, and the first name to appear on both lists would be offered the job. Wellington listed his in order of preference. Tim listed his alphabetically. Either way, Jan van Duser of the personnel department in the NFL office was the only name to appear on both lists. He turned the job down. He didn't have the appetite to get in the middle of a family free-for-all.

Finally, on February 8, 1979, it all exploded inside Giants Stadium. Wellington called a press conference. It was held in the press room on the ground floor of the stadium. The room was dreary, had no windows, and appropriately was called the Dungeon by the writers covering the team. There was an overflow media crowd jammed into the room. Wellington announced he was asserting his authority as president of the team to hire a coach, and he would address the GM opening at a later date. Tim stood in the back angry and horrified. The smoke coming out of his ears created a thick cloud above the stadium.

After Wellington finished outlining his plan, all hell broke loose. Tim quickly walked to the podium, not wanting the media to disperse. Wellington had zero interest in hearing Tim's rebuttal and exited out the back door of the press room and took the elevator one flight up to his office. "I want to have a winner," Tim said. "Well wants to have a winner—his way. Well's way has had us in the cellar the last fifteen years."

Reflecting on that moment after nearly a decade had passed, Tim said, "All of our wash came out in public."

Six days later, on Valentine's Day, George Young was announced as the Giants general manager at a press conference at Gallaghers Steakhouse in midtown Manhattan in the Theater District. The two Maras hardly kissed and made up on such a romantic day, but at least they had their man. The story of the path that led them to Young has never been told accurately until now.

To the day he died in 1995 from Hodgkin's disease at the age of fifty-nine, Tim may never have known how his uncle conspired behind his back with Rozelle to get Young hired. The story the Giants dispensed at the time was that after the dueling press conferences, Rozelle made the recommendation to the Maras to hire Young, who had worked in player personnel for Don Shula in Baltimore and Miami. Young interviewed with Bill Walsh to run the 49ers front office while he coached the team, but it was a lateral move, and Young wasn't interested. He wanted to be the decision maker. Ernie Accorsi, a future Giants GM and at the time the Colts assistant GM, was offered the job earlier the same day but said no. Instead, Walsh hired McVay, who had just been fired by the Giants.

Rozelle was hailed as hero for working through family politics and putting the Giants on the track to success by recommending Young. But that's not how it happened. The real story, according to John Mara:

Wellington knew any recommendation he made on his own to Tim would be rejected out of hand simply because of their relationship. They were pulling hard in different directions. But there are heroes to this story. Gifford, the Giants legend, and Tom Scott, who played linebacker for the Giants from 1959 to 1964, each recommended Young to their friend Wellington Mara. Young played high school football with Scott and asked him to contact Wellington Mara, which started the process.

Wellington was one of Rozelle's confidants, and the Giants had played a crucial role in growing the NFL into the financial behemoth it is today. In 1962, the Giants unselfishly agreed to share the revenue from the CBS network television broadcasts of their games, splitting it equally among the fourteen teams, even to smaller markets such as Green Bay. The precedent is still in effect today, and it has helped turn the league into the most popular TV product in America. The impact of the financial decision by the Giants to promote competitive balance was never lost on Rozelle, who was just two years into his twenty-nine-year term as commissioner.

During the GM search, Wellington told Rozelle that Young came highly recommended from Gifford and Scott, but if he brought his name to Tim, he had no chance of getting his approval. He requested Rozelle instead present Young's name as if it was his own suggestion. Rozelle did as asked and encouraged Wellington and Tim to hire Young. Uncle and nephew agreed and gave Young full control of the football operation. It was the most important hire in the history of the franchise.

Young managed to get along with both Maras, holding weekly meetings in a conference room every Wednesday, with the two owners communicating with each other through Young. He was adept at juggling the relationships and executing his more important plan: turning the Giants into winners. It was still hard to ignore the noise: Wellington and Tim had a fight over tickets shortly after Young was hired. Their suites at Giants Stadium were side by side and separated by a glass wall. They put up window coverings so they didn't have to see each other. They didn't speak to each other again until the final year of Tim's life in 1995 when Gifford negotiated a truce. They spoke about the Giants and family, and they each certainly had regrets.

"They hadn't been communicating," Gifford told the *New York Times*. "They had totally different lifestyles."

In a statement, Wellington Mara said, "A death in the family is a very personal thing. I hope people respect my privacy at this time."

Young had the Giants in the playoffs in three years. They won their first Super Bowl in his eighth season and another four years later. It was an impressively quick turnaround in the pre–free agency era. Tim decided in 1991 to sell his family's half of the team. He wanted $75 million. Wellington had right of first refusal but didn't have the resources to buy out Tim's 50 percent. Cleveland Browns owner Art Modell helped pair New York businessman Robert Tisch, the owner of the

Loews Corporation, with Tim Mara. Between the time they agreed on the price and the sale closing, the Giants won Super Bowl XXV. Tisch remarked that Tim never changed any of the terms. Surely, the price could have increased with the second Super Bowl title.

Despite the turmoil in the family, Tim was an honorable man, and Wellington Mara was the most respected man in the league. Tim was close to Parcells, who considered him an ally. On the day after the Giants beat Washington in the NFC Championship Game to advance to their first Super Bowl, an elderly couple was sitting in the team's lobby at the Giants Stadium office with tears flowing freely down their faces. They were longtime season ticket holders but were not selected in the Giants lottery to buy tickets for Super Bowl XXI. They had come to the office to plead their case but were told by the receptionist nothing could be done. So they went back to sit in the thick leather chairs a few feet away and cried.

I entered the lobby for a scheduled interview with Tim Mara and saw the heartbroken couple. They related their story. When Mara came out to walk me to his office, I told him about the two Giants fans. We went to his office, he opened his desk drawer, took out two tickets from the personal allotment he had purchased and went to visit with the couple. He handed them the tickets and instructed them to leave a check with the receptionist. The tickets were $75 each. The couple cried. It was such a kind act from a man not many knew about beyond fighting with his uncle at the press conference in 1979. Tim Mara made me promise I would not write about it. Perhaps he was concerned if the story went public fans would inundate him with their own heartfelt stories or line up in the lobby. He might have just wanted to remain relatively anonymous, as he had since Young was hired. I kept my promise until the day Tim died. In writing his obituary, I thought it was an important story for people to know about him. About a week later, I received a thank-you letter from his sister, Maura.

Tisch and Wellington admired and respected each other and were a good team. They died three weeks apart in the fall of 2005. Tisch, on his deathbed, cried when he was informed Wellington had passed away.

Their sons John Mara (he joined the team full time in 1991) and Steve Tisch have taken over for their fathers and enjoy an excellent relationship. Wellington and Tim are buried near each other in the family plot at Gate of Heaven Cemetery in Hawthorne, New York. Their names are on the tombstone with the names of Wellington's father Tim and his brother Jack, who was Tim's father.

IN 2022, THE Giants were valued by Forbes at $6 billion. If the Mara family's portion is a comparatively modest $3 billion—that's still a nice return on the elder Tim Mara's initial $500 investment, if they ever sell the team.

The Giants were started by a family, are now run by two families, and have always considered themselves one big family. "Once a Giant, Always a Giant," is their way of saying they take care of their own. Eli Manning added to the sentiment by closing his retirement press conference in January 2020, after playing his entire sixteen-year career with Big Blue: "Once a Giant, Always a Giant, Only a Giant."

Always a Giant?

As close knit as the '86 team is—perhaps more so than any other group of Giants—some members haven't felt the family love.

Pepper Johnson, Maurice Carthon, and William Roberts went on to become assistant coaches in the NFL, but the Giants never offered any of them jobs. Their Giants connections did help them with other teams, though. Johnson worked fourteen years for Bill Belichick in New England; Carthon worked a total of nine years for Parcells with the Patriots, Jets, and Cowboys; and Roberts worked one year for Parcells with the Jets. But not one member of the 1986 Giants, the most cherished of their Super Bowl teams, ever worked for the organization in coaching or in a front office role. Carl Banks, Harry Carson, and Karl Nelson have worked for the Giants on the broadcast side.

"Now, I'm not saying Lawrence wanted to coach, but others did," Roberts said. "They never really stepped out to any of us who started the championship run who wanted to coach."

When the Giants went through what's been referred to as the "wilderness years," when they were one of the worst teams in the NFL from the mid-'60s through the entirety of the '70s, Wellington Mara was criticized for attaching himself to former players such as Robustelli and Webster and scouts who were true blue even if not the most qualified for the job. When Young was hired, he frowned on hiring ex-Giants unless they had the credentials. He was determined to avoid the same path that had led the Giants into trouble.

After the two disastrous years of Ray Handley in 1991–1992 following Parcells, the Giants hired Reeves. He had no Giants ties other than having been interviewed by Wellington Mara. Once Tom Coughlin and Cowboys defensive coordinator Dave Wannstedt turned Young down, he reluctantly hired Reeves, fired by the Broncos, after a big push from Wellington Mara. Reeves had full control in Denver, and Young thought he wouldn't be able to adapt to the Giants' structure with Young in charge. He was right. Their relationship went sour after just one season. As the '86 Giants began to retire, Reeves was the head coach and had no connection to the players other than being on the losing sideline in Super Bowl XXI. "Dan Reeves came through and the rest is history," Roberts said. "He didn't have Giants blood in him."

After Reeves was fired after four seasons, Young hired Jim Fassel, who was the offensive coordinator for Handley. He was not around for either of the first two Super Bowls, and although he was on the staff for two years with Carthon, Roberts, and Johnson still playing on the team, they were not his guys. Coughlin replaced Fassel in 2004, and too much time had passed since he worked for Parcells from 1988 to 1990 as the wide receivers coach for him to have any allegiance to past Giants. By then Johnson was with Belichick, Carthon was with Parcells, and Roberts had gotten out of coaching.

"It's kind of a tricky area because you can't force a head coach and say, 'Hey, these guys were great former players of ours and they want to get into coaching, too,'" John Mara said. "George was very much against that sort of thing. It had to be all on merit. The former players are embraced as far as our feelings for them. We have alumni weekend every year, and most of those guys are invited back, and a lot of them do come back. But there are very limited jobs you can offer people in an organization, and if you start offering those jobs to every alumnus that was interested, that wouldn't work out very well."

The Giants do a nice job inviting players back each year and supplying them with two game tickets. The players are responsible for their travel and hotel, but the Giants attempt to offset that by arranging paid player appearances for a couple of thousand dollars. Players who have remained in the area are offered opportunities throughout the course of the season to shake hands and tell stories in suites with season ticket holders during games. Many of the Giants who went on to play for other teams say those clubs do not include the alumni on a regular basis like the Giants.

Wellington Mara's loyalty behind the scenes endeared him to players from multiple generations. Prior to the 1987 season, starting right tackle Karl Nelson was diagnosed with Hodgkin's disease. Nelson was scheduled for radiation and chemotherapy. The owners and players union were locked in a nasty stare-down in negotiations for a collective bargaining agreement. The second players' strike in six years was inevitable. Part of the 1982 CBA stated that the owners would cut off health insurance for the players on August 31 if there was not a new deal in place. If the players wanted health insurance, they could sign up for COBRA or opt into a plan set up by the NFL Players Association.

The players went on strike following the second game of the season. It lasted twenty-four days, less than half the fifty-seven days of the 1982 strike, but at the time there was no way of knowing whether it would last two weeks, two months, or wipe out the rest of the season. No time is good to be informed of a cancer diagnosis, but the timing was particularly troublesome for Nelson. He was undergoing radiation treatment at Memorial Sloan Kettering on the East Side of Manhattan five mornings a week for six weeks. On Sundays, the Giants kept him involved by adding him to their radio broadcasts as an analyst. When he was going through the chemotherapy treatments, there were three times he needed to stay in the hospital because his blood counts were low. The Giants paid to upgrade him to a private room and provide him with limousine service to bring him back and forth to the hospital.

"Whatever I needed, I got," he said. "Anything I needed, they were there."

But they did even more. Young called Nelson into his office and told him the Giants wanted to keep paying him his salary of $242,500 during the strike. All they wanted in return was a small favor. "We just ask that you don't be on the picket line," Young said. "And you don't say anything bad in the papers." Nelson went to the next union meeting and explained what the Giants wanted to do for him. "Everybody said, 'Yeah, absolutely, go ahead,'" Nelson said. "I was probably the only guy in the league that got sixteen game checks that year."

Nelson believed there was one reason he was paid.

"Because it was the Giants," he said. "Because it was Wellington Mara."

Nelson missed the entire 1987 season and came back to play the next year. Toward the end of the 1988 season, the cancer returned, which ended his career. He was treated again and was back in the radio booth from 1989 to 1994. He started Nelson Retirement Solutions, in the financial services field. He's also passionate about his volunteer work for Adopt-a-Soldier Platoon, which sends care packages to the military overseas and helps with care for the wounded when they return. Nelson got divorced and remarried around 2011, and his second wife's older son was serving in Afghanistan. The nonprofit organization sent him a package with three coffee makers, candy, and cigars. "He was the hit of the camp," Nelson said. That led him to get involved in the nonprofit organization, chairing their charity dinner.

He had his final cancer treatment in June 1989 and goes for checkups every six months. In 2017, he was diagnosed with two herniated discs and had two separate surgeries. He was about to have his third when a new doctor determined the muscle atrophy was a residual effect from the radiation nearly thirty years earlier. The doctor informed Nelson the first two surgeries were not necessary and instead he's worked hard at the gym strengthening the muscles that are still working well. "I can play golf," he said. "I just can't play two days in a row because the muscles in my back get too tired and my swing goes to hell."

The radiation was essential to rid him of the Hodgkin's and save his life. He's not complaining about having to deal with the radiation all these years later causing him aches and pains. Former Giants Doug Kotar and John Tuggle died from cancer, and Dan Lloyd was diagnosed with cancer. Although studies failed to connect the dots on whether it could have been an environmental issue at Giants Stadium, which was built on swamp and landfill, Nelson is not stressing over any connection.

"It doesn't matter what it was caused from," he said. "It is what it is."

———

PARCELLS RELEASED PHIL McConkey after the 1988 season, and he played for the Cardinals and Chargers in 1989 and then retired. After the '89 season, Parcells moved Romeo Crennel from special teams coach to defensive line and promoted Mike Sweatman from assistant special teams coach to special teams coach. That created an opening on his staff.

McConkey's phone rang shortly after he retired, and it was Parcells.

"I don't know what the fuck he wants," he said.

Parcells told McConkey, "As head coach of the team, my responsibility is to get the best possible guy qualified to take this role. You're it. So, as the head coach of the New York Giants, I'm offering you the job as assistant special teams coach."

He then repeated what he would later tell Bavaro after his summer with the Jets. "As your friend, I'm advising you not to take it," he said.

Long hours and low salary? Not very appealing. McConkey turned it down and decided to give politics a shot. He grew up in Buffalo, and former Bills quarterback and future congressman Jack Kemp was his boyhood idol. Kemp got him interested in a political career. McConkey ran for an open seat in the Twelfth Congressional District in New Jersey in 1990 and lost in the Republican primary. He received 12,925 votes (30.8 percent) and lost by 2,909 votes. "If I had run again, I would have won," he said. "I definitely would have been a congressman at some point—or maybe more. It wasn't the life for me. The biggest part was you're constantly fundraising, you're constantly asking people for money. I'm good at a lot of things. I'm not good at that."

When players are heading home for the day, coaches are ordering in dinner. It takes complete dedication to make the transition from playing to coaching. The great players who made life-changing money in the NFL want no part of lower-paying coaching positions. "Even marginal guys like me don't go back and do that," McConkey said. "You're a gopher as an assistant special teams coach. You're brand new and working twenty-five hours a day. It's brutal."

Mark Bavaro was offered a position on the Giants coaching staff in 1991 by Ray Handley after he took over for Parcells. Bavaro had been one of the Giants' best players in Super Bowl XXV in 1990 despite playing on a knee that would need bone graft surgery soon after the season. The next summer before camp, the Giants flunked Bavaro on the physical, and Young offered him only the $60,000 injury protection benefit when he was scheduled to make a career-high $750,000. Bavaro asked for $375,000, half of the money, while he rehabbed. If he was able to play in 1992, he would be paid the other half. If he couldn't play, the Giants would owe him nothing. Young said no. The Giants were hit with a backlash from the media for mistreating Bavaro, and Wellington Mara stepped in and offered him $315,000 with the other $60,000 coming in the injury protection benefit that was part of the collective bargaining agreement. Bavaro said, "I loved Mr. Mara and he apologized" for how Young treated him, "but I was hurt after everything I gave to the Giants. Just buying me off with fucking money and still sending me away." His pride almost convinced him to leave the money on the table, but he changed his mind after his mentor and former teammate Don Hasselbeck told him to take $10,000 out of the bank in small bills, lay the cash on the floor of his house, and then think how thirty-seven times that much would look.

Message received.

The next day, Bavaro returned to Mara's hotel suite. He knocked on the door, and Mara appeared. "Okay, I'll take the money," he said.

Handley wanted Bavaro to tutor third-year tight end Howard Cross and some of the other young players. He knew his knee would not allow him to play in 1991, but he asked Handley if he could rehab at the Giants facilities during the time he wasn't coaching with an agreement he could attempt a comeback with the Giants in 1992 if he was healthy. Handley checked with his bosses.

"No, that's not going to happen," Handley said.

Bavaro still wanted to play if his knee checked out. He had already decided to sell his house in Chatham, and he rejected Handley's offer. He moved back to the Boston area. His wife Susan, who had completed two years at Seton Hall Law School, transferred to Harvard to finish up her studies. Bavaro was able to return to the field in 1992 and played one year for Belichick in Cleveland, followed by two years in Philadelphia.

Pepper Johnson was different from McConkey and Bavaro. He was committed to coaching. A few years after Coughlin was hired as the Giants head coach, Johnson called him about a job. Johnson already had won three Super Bowls as a member of Belichick's defensive staff with the Patriots but thought it was important for his career to prove himself in another system. Johnson said Coughlin told him he didn't have any vacancies. That was disappointing. He stayed in New England and made it to two more Super Bowls, both losses to Coughlin and the Giants. By the end of the 2013 season, Johnson had been passed over many times by Belichick when the defensive coordinator's job opened up with the Patriots. They mutually decided it was time for him to move on. He took a job as Doug Marrone's defensive line coach with the Bills.

"My goal and my dream was that I wanted to be able to do this on my own and not under the shadow of Bill Belichick," Johnson said.

"I wanted to see if I could call the defenses in the league. I wanted to not be up under Coach Belichick."

Following the 2014 season, Coughlin fired defensive coordinator Perry Fewell. Immediately, the overwhelming favorite to get the job was Steve Spagnuolo, who had been Coughlin's defensive coordinator on the Super Bowl XLII team that knocked off the undefeated Patriots.

As part of the process, Coughlin requested to interview Johnson. He was anxious to rise above being position coach, and this was his first interview for defensive coordinator. "When I started coaching, I thought, man, if there was ever a dream job, it would be to go back and coach with the Giants," Johnson said. "I didn't think I could ever fulfill that dream until Coughlin said to come to New Jersey and he would interview me for a job. I felt like Reggie Jackson in October. There was no doubt in my mind that I wasn't getting ready to slap it out of the park."

He didn't go deep. He hit a lazy fly ball to center.

"How do you do an interview with anybody where you know more than what they do?" Johnson said. "This is no way of disrespecting Coach Coughlin, but the questions that he was asking me about defense, I don't know if he understood my answers."

Coughlin was grilling him on what schemes he would design to stop Chip Kelly's high-powered fastbreak offense in Philadelphia. Kelly didn't accept Coughlin's offer to become the Giants offensive quality control coach in 2006, when Kelly was the offensive coordinator at the University of New Hampshire. In his years as the Oregon head coach and especially his first season coaching the Eagles in 2013, Kelly's innovative offense was hard to stop. Johnson presented his plan to Coughlin. He walked out of the interview hoping he did well enough to convince Coughlin to hire him or at least have a follow-up conversation. "I had kind of a mixed emotion," Johnson said. "I thought he was just picking my brain. I really did."

Coughlin, as expected, hired Spagnuolo in what turned out to be his final year as the Giants head coach. Marrone opted out of his Buffalo contract after Johnson's first season with the Bills after he was led to believe the Jets were going to hire him to replace Rex Ryan. Instead, Jets owner Woody Johnson changed his mind and hired Todd Bowles, and Ryan replaced Marrone in Buffalo. That left Marrone without a job—he later signed on as assistant head coach and offensive line coach in Jacksonville—and Johnson hoping to at least hang onto his job in Buffalo.

Johnson thought he had an understanding with Ryan that he would be retained on his new staff if he didn't get the coordinator job with the Giants. After Coughlin called Johnson with the bad news, he was preparing to drive back to Buffalo from his home in New England to meet with Ryan and finalize his responsibilities. Instead, a member of the media aware of Johnson's travel plans called to read him a press release that had just been issued by the Bills to announce Ryan's staff. Johnson was not included.

He was unemployed.

Johnson was never shy about speaking his mind during his playing days with the Giants, whether it was about what was happening on the field or with his contract. He was an excellent player, knew the game like a coach, but his personality was not for everybody. "I was a rebel," he said. "I can't just say it looking at it in hindsight. I knew it back then. And I knew some of the things I was doing and saying were dangerous. But I couldn't be me if I didn't. I don't know how I would have lived with myself."

He was out of work a couple weeks when Bowles hired him to be the Jets defensive line coach. He was fired after two seasons and never worked in the NFL again. He spent one season each as a defensive assistant in three spring leagues and as the head coach at IMG Academy in Florida.

"I'm done with coaching," he said.

Carthon also was disappointed the Giants never asked him to join their coaching staff. The closest any Carthon came to being hired by the Giants is when Mo's son Ran, a personnel executive with the 49ers, interviewed for the general manager job that went to Joe Schoen in 2022. Ran Carthon was hired one year later as the Tennessee Titans general manager. When Johnson lived with Mo Carthon in Jonesboro in 2019 during his one year coaching in Memphis in the Alliance league, they talked a lot about how neither of them was ever offered a coaching job with the team where they won two Super Bowls.

"We never knew the reason why," Carthon said.

———

JOHN MARA IS sensitive to the financial, physical, and mental health needs of his former players. The Giants plan to resurrect a program started before the pandemic in 2020 offering internships to their retired players. The players are rotated through different departments, either on the football or business side, to help determine whether they want to pursue it as a career. Many have never had a job outside of playing and have no idea about the inner workings of a football organization after just dealing with the general manager, coaches, teammates, and trainers during their career.

"It's not going to help a lot of people, but if we could just help a couple of guys a year to figure out if this is the direction they want to go in, it would be well worth our effort, whatever the expenses," Mara said. "But it's not necessarily meant for guys in their fifties and sixties but for the twenty-eight-year-old guy whose career just ended and is thinking: Now what do I do with myself?"

Mara inherited his compassion for his players from his father. Even so, it makes sense that the Giants don't advertise all the good work they do behind the scenes. They are a business, and it would be very costly to bail out every former player from a tough situation. But they are open to listening.

It's the players from the era of the '86 Giants who need the most help. NFL salaries were radically different, and many needed offseason jobs to help pay the bills. If the Giants find out a player is in trouble, they try to help behind the scenes, as they have with Brad Benson. Mara has tried to be attentive to the needs of his former players. When he was informed in 2007 that Webster, who has since passed away, didn't have the money to buy an electronic lift to raise him in his wheelchair into his car and couldn't afford health insurance to defray the cost, Mara made arrangements to take care of it for him. "He's more than a former player," Mara said at the time. "He's been a good family friend for many years. I've known him for almost my entire life."

The stories have not improved over the years. "I know there are some guys with challenges," Mara said. "We're definitely concerned. For those we aren't aware of, I just wish they'd reach out. Maybe there is some sort of help we can find for them because there are resources out there that the NFL makes available that we'd be willing to make available."

One player on the '86 Giants who played more than ten years in the league said he took his pension early when he was fifty-five years old. "My understanding is football players die at an earlier rate," he said. His monthly check is $2,600, considerably lower than if he had waited. The legacy benefit that was negotiated in the 2011 and 2020 collective bargaining agreements gives players with a minimum three credited seasons about an extra $300 per month for each season they played. The improvements were put in motion with Harry Carson's compelling Hall of Fame speech in 2006 imploring the league not to forget the retired players who set the foundation for what the league had become and now need help. "If I had to do it over again, I would have said more," he said.

Until Carson opened his mouth, it had been a struggle for retired players to convince the NFL Players Association leadership to put up more of a fight for them. The union always prioritized current players, whose union dues pay the salaries of the union executives. Carson was disgusted with Gene Upshaw, the former Hall of Fame guard for the Oakland Raiders, who was the NFLPA executive director for twenty-five years until his death in 2008. Upshaw angered retired players with a comment he made about them in 2007 to the *Charlotte Observer*. "The bottom line is I don't work for them," he said. "They don't hire me and they can't fire me. They can complain about me all day long. They can have their opinion. But the active players have the vote. That's who pays my salary."

Health insurance is just as important to retired players as their pension benefits. Maybe even more important. The '86 Giants didn't play long enough to receive the current benefit of five years of post-retirement insurance coverage for vested players with at least three years of service that was part of the 2006 CBA. Almost all of the Giants were out of the league by 1995, which qualified them for only one year of insurance. The insurance increased to two years and then three years in subsequent seasons before it finally went to five. Many players experience health issues or need hip, shoulder, and knee replacement surgery in their fifties and sixties, and the league now has different funds and networks for all retired players to help defray the cost. The improvements for retired players in the two most recent CBAs were negotiated by DeMaurice Smith, who succeeded Upshaw after he died.

"I think players should have lifelong health care," Carson said. "Five years after you leave football, you still feel relatively fine. When you get down the road, your body starts to break down."

The physical, mental and financial issues of retired players are heartbreaking, but the '86 Giants rallying around their teammates in need is heartwarming. Life after football can be overwhelming, but the brotherhood of the '86 Giants serves as a safety net.

"Harry has a genuine concern for each of the guys he played with and really does consider them brothers," Mara said. "If one of them is facing difficult issues, he's the first guy to stand up and try to rally others for support. Phil Simms is like that, too. And George Martin. Just good human beings in addition to being great players."

"Harry is an amazing guy, an amazing friend," Marshall said. "I love him to death and will love him to death to the day we die."

"When you win a championship, you create a bond, and that bond is with you forever," Carson said. "We all bleed the same blood and it's blue. We look out for one another. We love one another. We are all brothers."

Carson went above and beyond for wide receiver Lionel Manuel. One night during training camp, Carson heard him arguing with his girlfriend on the pay phone in the hallway of the dormitory. It turned out she was pregnant, and Carson surmised Manuel was not happy about it. Carson happened to be friends with the woman. Before the baby was born, Carson told her, "If you need somebody to help you get through this, let me know." Before she gave birth, Carson said Manuel was engaged to another woman.

Early on a Sunday morning in the offseason, Carson's phone rang at his home in New Jersey.

"I'm looking for Harry Carson," the man said.

"This is Harry," he said.

"I'm the doctor in the labor room at Mt. Sinai Hospital and there is a woman asking for you," he said.

It was 7 a.m. Carson jumped in his car, put on his flashers and made it to the hospital as fast as he could. He went right to the maternity unit and walked into the delivery room. He introduced himself, then washed his hands as the doctor and the labor room nurses looked at him like a deadbeat dad.

"I got one thing to say," Carson said. "This is not my child."

He then assisted in the birth. In the small world department, the ob-gyn was from Baltimore. His high school teacher was George Young.

Simms hasn't played stand-in in the delivery room, but he has helped teammates in many ways behind the scenes. "He's done things nobody knows about where he's helped people without anything in return," Oates said. "I know of one situation where he was burned for it. But it won't prevent him from helping other guys."

Two weeks before the 1983 draft, the Giants traded defensive end Gary Jeter to the Los Angeles Rams. They replaced him by selecting Marshall from LSU in the second round. Jeter had an apartment in Secaucus he was anxious to rent, and Taylor introduced them. Marshall took Jeter's job and apartment. Training camp arrived before Marshall had a chance to move in, and he had all his belongings in a U-Haul. Taylor invited him to park in his driveway at his home until the Giants returned from camp.

The Giants had a tradition each Saturday during the season requiring first-round picks to bring in doughnuts and second-round picks to bring in coffee and juice. "Guys like Phil and Lawrence showed us the definitive landscape how things work," Marshall said.

He fulfilled his obligations his rookie year and later educated Pepper Johnson, one of the Giants second-round picks in 1986. That helped bring them together as friends. By then, Marshall was living in an apartment complex in East Rutherford. Marshall helped Johnson find a place to live in the same development.

Little things make teammates play harder for each other on Sunday.

Big things make the bond unbreakable.

One Giant said he has written checks for over $50,000 to teammates who need assistance. He also said a teammate came to him distraught that his mother was on the verge of losing her house, and he helped out by loaning a substantial amount of money to resolve issues with the mortgage.

"Winning the Super Bowl has a lot to do with it. Winning has a lot to do with everything," Jim Burt said. "You're spending six or seven months a year together for eleven or twelve years. For most people, it's the peak of their life. The only thing that I can think of that is way more is the military. Guys in the military got each other's back, and they're actually fighting for each other's lives. Football has got nothing to do with that, but you need to have a brotherhood to win."

When Carson discovered Burt had not scheduled annual medical checkups for the first ten years after he retired, he ordered him to make a doctor's appointment for a comprehensive exam. Burt felt fine but held off on a doctor's visit, fearing a medical issue would be discovered. "It made me feel good that Harry cared about me," Burt said. Carson and his wife picked Burt up at his home. Why did he avoid going? "I just didn't want to deal with it," he said. "Harry got me to do it. I said, 'Okay, you come get me, I'll do it.'"

Burt asked Carson to go with him again for his appointment the following year and then committed to going every year on his own.

Burt is paying it forward by encouraging reluctant teammates from the '86 Giants to get regular checkups. Carson is haunted by memories of his close friend Brad Van Pelt, a former teammate, whom he was unable to convince to see a doctor regularly after his playing days ended with the Browns in 1986. Van Pelt was a heavy drinker and partier and died from a heart attack in 2009. He was only fifty-seven years old. Carson is determined not to allow abstaining from doctor's visits be the precursor to the death of any other teammate. He is so well respected that players from other teams often call him for advice.

In addition to Carson driving him to the doctor, Burt insisted on one other condition: Carson had to accompany him into the examining room. Carson said he remained even when the doctor checked Burt's prostate by inserting his finger into his rectum.

"I turned and didn't watch," Carson said.

Sometimes loyalty means looking away, too.

Burt laughed when he heard Carson's version.

"That's bullshit," he said. "Harry wasn't sitting in the room when they stuck their finger in there. He's making that shit up. Now he's going too far. No way I wanted him in the room when they are sticking anything up my ass. That's so funny."

All of Burt's body parts and organs checked out fine.

"That's just football players, men in general, have a tendency not to take care of themselves as they should," Carson said. "As a result, a lot of guys keel over."

Parcells was always tough on Burt, an undrafted free agent nose tackle. He was the ultimate try-hard guy. There was a great deal of friction in their relationship based on their competitiveness. But when Burt found out Parcells was going for shoulder replacement surgery in Manhattan twenty-five years after he last played for him, he insisted Parcells stay at his house in New Jersey rather than at a hotel the night before the surgery. Burt took Parcells into the city for the surgery, picked him up days later, and then drove him the 180 miles back to his house in Saratoga.

The morning of the surgery, Parcells was antsy and up at five o'clock and pacing in Burt's house.

"I don't know what the hell he was doing," Burt said laughing.

Parcells grabbed his overnight bag, and they drove into Manhattan. When he returned to the hospital the day Parcells was released, there were a couple of doctors in Parcells's room at the time Burt walked in. They were giving him instructions how to get his clothes on and perform simple tasks to deal with his new shoulder during the recuperation period.

"Parcells is giving these guys a hard time," Burt said. "He's breaking their balls."

Burt was taking it all in. It brought him back to training camp. Parcells was sparring with his doctors just like he did with his players.

"Guys, why are you telling him all this stuff?" Burt said.

"We want him to be able to function when he gets home," one doctor said.

"He's never going to make it home," Burt said.

The doctors and Parcells looked at Burt. Their eyes asked, *What the hell is he talking about?*

"I'm driving him on the New York State Thruway," Burt said. "Do you know how many cliffs there are over there? After everything he did to me, I'm throwing his ass off the side."

Parcells was just coming down from the post-surgery drugs. "He looked at me like, 'I'm not getting into the car with this guy,'" Burt said. "I started laughing my ass off. I could see how serious he was. He thinks I'm actually going to get him back for all he did to me."

Burt, of course, drove him safely home for his recovery.

"I love the guy," Burt said.

The brotherhood of the 1986 Super Bowl champion New York Giants is as strong as ever.

EPILOGUE

O nce a Giant and, to varying degrees, always a Giant.

They will always have 1986. They will always have one another.

That's the beautiful thing about sports.

The '86 Giants came from all over the country. One came from Mexico. From big-time college football programs and from small schools and HBCUs. The forty-five-man roster for Super Bowl XXI on January 25, 1987, had twenty-eight African American players and seventeen white players, but the consensus was the locker room was one color.

Big Blue.

When reunions or memorabilia shows bring the group together, it takes them right back to '86, and they start acting like kids in their midtwenties instead of fathers and grandfathers in their fifties, sixties, and seventies.

Their bond is real. They are there for one another. They take care of one another.

"This team here is maybe the greatest laboratory for human behavior that I have ever witnessed," Bill Parcells said in an ESPN story in 2011 at the twenty-fifth reunion. "I wish society had a chance to witness the interaction of all this conglomeration of people that we had on this team, from all different parts of the country. Sensitivity isn't tolerated. There are no secrets. When we all got together in that room, it was like nothing changed."

Life does go on, however.

Only the fortunate few left the Giants on their own terms. Even Phil Simms, the MVP of the Super Bowl, had the decision made for him. In real time, they become numb to the hellos and goodbyes of roster upheaval. "Guys get cut left and right," Mark Bavaro said. "They come and go, and sometimes you don't even notice they're gone."

The goal for my research was to discover how life after football has treated the '86 Giants and to reveal how their bond became so strong and why it will last a lifetime.

The love-hate relationship with Parcells motivated them. The laboratory experiment in the locker room worked to perfection. Teammates worried about Lawrence Taylor; tried to avoid being victimized by practical jokers Simms, Jim Burt, Mark Collins, and Bart Oates; were mesmerized by the life lessons taught by Harry Carson and George Martin, blown away by Mark Bavaro's toughness and Bill Belichick's brains, and jealous of Sean Landeta's way with women.

In life after football, becoming successful, happy, and healthy are the goals. Nobody has gone three for three.

Bavaro was the most compelling and emotional interview I conducted. That might surprise those who remember Mark from his playing days as unusually shy, but that just wasn't the right time in his life to open up. When he was telling me the story of his final days with the Giants, when George Young wasn't doing right by him with the money, he talked about a twelve-year-old boy with cancer he had befriended. The boy called up a radio show criticizing the Giants for not taking care of his hero. Cancer took his life. Bavaro had to stop several times telling this anecdote. His voice cracked. He couldn't get out the words.

This was the Bavaro the Giants fans adored but didn't know.

As much fun as it was reconnecting with the players and coaches, I was really saddened to hear Bavaro, Leonard Marshall, and Curtis McGriff explain how they considered suicide to overcome issues that may have been caused or at least exacerbated by football. Bobby Johnson's life was literally in the gutter; he was homeless and sleeping on a park bench in Nashville. One freezing night he was one step from jumping off a bridge into the chilly waters of the Cumberland River. And Carson's story about his plan to drive off the Tappan Zee Bridge into the Hudson River was really numbing. I drove across that bridge hundreds of times before it was torn down.

My prior relationships with so many of the '86 Giants gave me a running start researching this book. They knew they could trust me. I really appreciate how forthcoming they were about the most sensitive experiences in their lives. In the more than four decades I spent covering the NFL, so many of my favorite people played for the '86 Giants.

———

I CAN STILL remember my first NFL game as a kid. It was 1968, and my father took me to Yankee Stadium to see the New York Giants play the Philadelphia Eagles. We sat in the bleachers behind one of the end zones, it was freezing, I drank a lot of hot chocolate, and the Giants won in a 7–6 *thriller*.

My father worked for CBS, and the second game I attended we had field passes and watched from behind the Giants bench. I couldn't see much with all the big guys standing on the sideline in front of me. The view was much better from the bleachers. It was a thrill to be at the stadium, especially because in those days, the home games were blacked out.

All the Giants needed to do to make the playoffs in 1970 was beat the Los Angeles Rams in the final game of the season at Yankee Stadium. My father was invited to a watch party (who knows what they called it in those days) at the CBS Broadcast Center on West Fifty-Seventh Street.

"Want to go?" he asked.

"Are you kidding me?" I said.

On the first series, Fran Tarkenton overthrew a deep pass to running back Tucker Frederickson down the right sideline—I can remember it like it was yesterday—for what would have been an easy touchdown. That was the game. The Giants lost 31–3.

My first job out of Syracuse was working for the Associated Press, and the Giants were the first NFL team I covered. Any allegiance I had as a kid was completely gone as soon as journalism became my profession. The Giants provided the first true test of my skills on deadline. I had dictated my story to the New York office of a mid-November game in 1978 and was counting down the seconds to the editor of a 17–12 victory for the Giants over the Eagles. The idea was to get the story on the wire the instant the game ended so that newspapers that also subscribed to UPI would use the AP story. My countdown started at thirty seconds, and I made it to twenty-five.

"Holy shit. Don't send that story yet," I said to the editor.

"What happened?" he said.

I told him to turn around to the television in the AP's Rockefeller Center office and watch the replay of Joe Pisarcik trying to hand off to Larry Csonka, instead of doing the only sensible thing and kneeling on the ball.

"Holy shit," the editor agreed.

He watched what I had seen live: the loose ball being scooped up by Eagles cornerback Herm Edwards and returned twenty-six yards for the winning touchdown with twenty seconds left. I dictated a new story in record time.

The play became a slice of NFL history. The Fumble.

I was at Giants Stadium the day the Giants brought in little-known first-round quarterback Phil Simms for a press conference a couple of days after shocking fans by taking him seventh overall in 1979. For some reason, one of the photographers asked Simms to sign his name on a chalkboard in the press room. Simms picked up the chalk with his left hand and signed. A cynical media person (not me) cracked, "Do the Giants know Simms is lefthanded?" He was righthanded but writes with his left hand. Simms is one of my all-time favorites. He was a great player, but I'm talking about as a person.

As I started on this project in the fall of 2021, I wondered, Would any of it have happened without Lawrence Taylor?

Full disclosure: I nearly cost the Giants the chance to draft him.

It was not my intention, of course, but I was the reason Taylor sent Giants coach Ray Perkins a telegram the day before the 1981 draft, warning the Giants not to take him.

The backstory: In the spring of '81, I had just been promoted to Giants beat writer by my sports editors Buddy Martin and Gene Williams after less than one year at the *New York Daily News*. The Giants were the second–most important sports beat at the newspaper behind the Yankees, and I was young and eager to make a name for myself in the tabloid wars. I had been around the Giants for two years for the AP.

As long as the Saints did as expected and drafted South Carolina running back George Rogers, the Heisman winner, with the first overall pick, then the Giants, who were picking second, were locked in on Taylor, a linebacker from North Carolina who could wreck a game with his size and speed, relentless attitude, and endless energy.

Bum Phillips was in his first year as the coach and general manager of the Saints in 1981 after he was fired as coach of the Houston Oilers. He envisioned Rogers doing for the Saints what Earl Campbell had done for him with the Oilers. There were twenty-eight teams in the NFL, and the Giants were lucky Phillips was in control of the only pick ahead of them. Dick Steinberg had been the Saints vice president of personnel but resigned after Phillips was hired. Steinberg said he would have drafted Taylor. But without Steinberg's influence, the Saints were thought to be the only team that would have drafted Rogers over Taylor.

As a result of knowing the Giants players from working at the AP, I had excellent sources. And they were chirping a few days before Taylor became a teammate.

One of the offensive veterans called me aside in the locker room and leaked that several defensive players were upset with the three-year, $1 million contract number they heard the Giants were going to give Taylor and were planning to boycott training camp if he signed for more than they were making—especially that much more. Several Rams actually carried through on a similar threat the previous summer and came back only when they were promised raises at the end of the season. I interviewed a handful of the Giants defensive veterans that day, and they confirmed they were angry and no-showing for training camp was on the agenda.

On the Sunday before the draft, the *Daily News* headline stretched across the top of the back page in big, bold letters read:

GIANTS VETERANS THREATEN WALKOUT

When I called Giants owner Wellington Mara for comment, he said, "My respect for you as a newspaper man has greatly diminished." I was twenty-six years old. I admired Mara, and his words disappointed me. It was not as if I was suggesting the players stage a boycott. I was reporting that his players were considering it. I've never been afraid to write stories that I knew would be unpopular and piss people off as long as I knew I was right. If I could be intimidated, then I was in the wrong business.

The Giants had not made the playoffs since 1963, had not won a playoff game since 1958, and were coming off a 4–12 season in which they gave up twenty-seven points a game, second worst to the Saints. GM George Young and Perkins likely would have welcomed a boycott and a chance to start over on defense, even though the strength of the team was linebackers Harry Carson, Brad Van Pelt, and Brian Kelley. Regardless, it would have been malpractice for them to pass on Taylor.

Defensive end Gary Jeter was the Giants highest-paid player in 1981 at $145,000, Van Pelt was making $130,000 coming off five straight Pro Bowls, and Carson was at $120,000. The draft was held on Tuesday, April 28. Taylor fired off a telegram to Perkins on Monday after hearing about my story from one day earlier. He did not want to play for the Giants if it meant walking into a hostile locker room, and it was clear to him it was hostile.

A few Giants reached out to Taylor the same day he wrote the telegram. They told him they were rooting for him to get all the money he could knowing it could help them in the future. Their issue was not with him but with the organization. That satisfied L.T.

Young was already scared the Saints were going to change their mind at the last minute and draft Taylor or trade the pick to the Cowboys. Much of Young's weekend was spent tracking down rumors Taylor was in Dallas or New Orleans or actually had visited both. He called hotels and airlines trying to find him. He was in North Carolina. If Taylor was off the board, the Giants would have taken Rogers, who led the NFL in rushing as a rookie.

Side note: There was a chalkboard in the media room at Giants Stadium. A couple of the guys kept a running total during the 1980 season of Rogers's yardage versus the Giants running backs'. Rogers ran for 1,781 yards in eleven games. The Giants ran for 1,586 yards in sixteen.

The 1981 draft got off to a rough start at the New York Sheraton. Commissioner Pete Rozelle was stuck in the hotel elevator for twenty minutes coming down to the ballroom, and then his microphone was not working. After the Saints selected Rogers, it took only fifteen seconds before Rozelle uttered the most impactful twelve words in Giants history: "The New York Giants first-round selection, Lawrence Taylor, linebacker, North Carolina."

Taylor apologized to Perkins for the telegram. Five hours later, he had arrived in New Jersey and was in his hotel room taking a nap. "I went to sleep around six. I was really tired," he said then. "Then I got up around 9:30 to watch television. They got a pretty good selection here. I watched *The Three Stooges.*"

New York offered more sophisticated culture than *The Three Stooges*, and Taylor didn't take long to find out. In fact, he found out way too much.

He signed a three-year, $600,000 contract, making him the highest-paid player in Giants history. He also received a $300,000 loan. Pretty soon, he didn't have time for *The Three Stooges* between football and getting acquainted with New York.

The course of Giants history and NFL history would have been vastly different if Young and Perkins didn't hold strong after Taylor's telegram. And if the Giants passed on him, it would've been the result of my story. Four decades later, it still amazes me how my story quoting a handful of disgruntled players could have cost the Giants the greatest defensive player in NFL history.

I covered the NFL on a day-to-day basis for the Associated Press, *Dallas Morning News*, *New York Daily News*, HBO's *Inside the NFL*, and the YES Network's *This Week in Football*, and this is my sixth book about the NFL, including *The Catch*, and the *New York Times* bestseller, *Brady vs. Manning*.

I've gotten to know hundreds and hundreds of players when they were in their twenties and stayed in touch with many who are now in their fifties, sixties, and seventies. Football is a brutal sport. How they are handling life after football is an important story to tell.

I initially came up with the idea to write this book while attending the Pro Football Hall of Fame induction in 2017. The day before the ceremony, the HOF had an event for the previous gold jacket recipients who had come back to Canton for the weekend. It struck me as I looked to the stage as the players assembled for a picture: Paul Hornung had a cane by his side. He had been diagnosed with dementia. Earl Campbell needed a walker to help him get back into his wheelchair. He had both of his knees replaced, endured five back surgeries, and overcame an addiction to painkillers. Jim Brown was walking with a cane. Gale Sayers was suffering from Alzheimer's disease. Tony Dorsett was experiencing memory loss issues and required a driver back home in Dallas to navigate the streets he's known since 1977.

The Hall of Famers' stories were crushing. I needed to know more.

═══

MY JOURNEY BEGAN at the most logical place: the captain's house. I first met Harry Carson in 1978 when he was twenty-five years old in his third season. I've stayed in touch with him regularly since his playing days ended. It was appropriate to have Carson set the table and give his insight into what the '86 Giants were all about. I spent a few hours with Carson. His wife Maribel was in and out doing errands, his dog Charley sat by his feet, and his bird was chirping.

Simms was honest and raw about his severe back issues that only his inner circle knew about when I visited him at his home in Franklin Lakes, New Jersey. It was sad listening to his desperation to deaden the pain with vodka and painkillers. His football career gave him so much and set him up for his long television career, but he paid the price. Phil is a great storyteller, and his recollection of his dinner with Billy Crystal and Phil McConkey two nights before the Super Bowl was entertaining. In fact, it was Simms who suggested that I get in touch with Crystal. From my HBO days, I have a friend, Ross Greenburg, who is close to Crystal, and he facilitated connecting me with Billy to reminisce about the dinner from his hilarious perspective.

I visited Mark Bavaro in his living room in Boxford, Massachusetts, and sat for more than two hours. "Mark must really like you," his wife Susan said. "He doesn't talk to anybody for two hours." I dropped by to see Leonard Marshall at his home in New Jersey, Carl Banks at his office in midtown Manhattan, and Phil McConkey in the lobby of a New York hotel when he was in town on a business trip from San Diego. I spoke to Bobby Johnson in Smyrna, Tennessee, years ago and again when he attended a 2022 Giants reunion at MetLife Stadium.

The most productive day was a morning-afternoon split double-header in Florida with Parcells and Taylor.

Parcells used to bark at me in press conferences when he thought I asked a stupid question—that was entirely possible. At his house in Tequesta, he gave me a tour of his office with all the memorabilia of his coaching career. After we wrapped up the interview, we walked out to his deck with a great view of the Intercoastal. It wasn't oceanfront property in Sea Girt, but it was very nice. In the afternoon, I drove twenty minutes to the Old Palm Golf Club in Palm Beach Garden for Joe Namath's celebrity golf tournament.

If there is a golf tournament with former athletes paired with rich people who pay lots of money to charity to play with them, it's a good bet No. 56 will be there. I scheduled one week ahead of the tournament to meet with Taylor after he finished his round. Namath arranged a lunch with an auction for his guests, and I figured when Taylor finished eating I would approach him.

I texted him to let him know where I was waiting.

No response.

I looked for him at the luncheon.

Didn't see him.

I walked out to the front of the club to the valet parking area and the attendant told me Taylor put his golf clubs in his car. Uh-oh. Did he leave? "All the players are putting their clubs in their cars and coming back in for the luncheon," he said. "None of them are leaving their things in the clubhouse." I felt better until he said, "But I didn't see Lawrence return."

Did he forget about me?

It took me back to two days before Christmas in 1998 when I set up an interview at Taylor's house in Upper Saddle River. It was about one month before the Hall of Fame vote, and he accepted my invitation to talk about what was going on in his life. I wanted his opinion about selectors who might be hesitant to vote for him because of his cocaine addiction even though the HOF mandates off-the-field issues are not to be considered. I showed up exactly on time, rang the doorbell, and nobody was home. I called his assistant; she tracked him down and promised he would be there within thirty minutes. I took a ride around the neighborhood and came back in twenty minutes, and his car was out front. He apologized for being late. Even though it was a frigid day, he was out on the golf course playing "an emergency nine," he said. Taylor was in a talkative mood and, of course, smoking a cigar. He spoke about recently completing a forty-eight-day stay at the Honesty House rehab facility in Sterling, New Jersey, and that he was still spending most nights and weekends at the center. The *Daily News* back page the next day had a picture of L.T. in his kitchen. The huge headline said, "LT Speaks." Inside with my stories was a picture of him enveloped in a cloud of cigar smoke. Taylor left a message on my answering machine at home the next day after he read the story and thanked me for treating him fairly.

Back to Florida. After the valet told me he had not seen Taylor after he went to the parking lot, I was not happy. I had arranged my time with Parcells so I could also meet with Taylor. I was not about to chase him all over South Florida.

I tried to call him.

No answer.

I texted him again.

No response.

I went back to the tent at the luncheon. Brooks Thomas, who used to work for the Jets in public relations, and his wife, Linda, organize the annual event for Namath. They knew I was there to meet with Taylor. Linda had already realized Taylor skipped the luncheon and called him on his cell and told him he had to turn around and come back to talk with me. She said I had come from New York to meet with him and he couldn't stand me up. He would be back in fifteen minutes, he told Linda.

Taylor's friend who drives him dropped the car off at the valet stand. Taylor once again apologized, this time for forgetting about our appointment. We walked to a veranda, sat down at a table, and he lit up a cigar. He looked healthy. He was happy.

"You know that ten years ago you never would have turned around and come back," I said to him.

"You're right," he said.

Parcells and Taylor in one day made this a very good day.

Not one player turned down my request for an interview. I really wanted to get Bill Belichick's perspective. I was never all that friendly with him when he was a Giants assistant. When I traveled to Cleveland to do an interview with him in his first training camp as the head coach of the Browns in 1991, he spoke to me while he was out of breath on the treadmill. He didn't want to talk before or after he worked out. I thought that was disrespectful.

We had minimal interaction in his three years with the Jets and during his early years in New England. I was very critical of him in the *Daily News* during the 2007 Spygate controversy, and as a result he wasn't all that nice to me when I tried to ask him questions in press conferences. Oh well, what can you do? Then, in January 2020, we sat next to each other for eight hours at a Hall of Fame meeting in Canton. It was going to be a very long day if we ignored each other. I broke the ice, and we had a fun time talking back and forth. I saw the other side of Belichick that his friends always told me existed, and we've kept in touch via email.

I contacted Bill when I started my research and asked whether I could come up and visit in Foxborough. Belichick rarely participates in book projects, so I wasn't sure how he would handle it. He told me his answers would be more comprehensive if he could think about the questions and email me his responses. That was better than a rejection and not as good as face to face, but it was a productive compromise. He was such a big part of the Giants success that I very much wanted his voice in the book. I sent Bill fifteen questions, and he answered with his typical depth. The document was nearly 2,500 words.

Belichick's love for the '86 Giants speaks to not only how these players and coaches feel about each other, but the love affair they had with the fans as they delivered the team's first Super Bowl title. Ask any Giants fan who has witnessed all four of their Super Bowl wins how they rank the accomplishments, and they will say the victory over the undefeated Patriots in Super Bowl XLII was the most thrilling, but it's the 1986 team—with L. T., Simms, Banks, Carson, Bavaro, Marshall, and the superstar coaching staff led by Parcells and Belichick—that will always occupy the number one spot in their hearts.

As the '86 Giants have grown old together and face the challenges of life after football, the brotherhood remains unbreakable, and that may be their greatest legacy of all.

ACKNOWLEDGMENTS

I want to thank my wife, Allison, for her unwavering support and most of all for not protesting my hostile takeover of the dining room to write this book when I got tired of working in my office. And who knew she was such a big football fan? On January 11, 1987, I was very comfortable sitting in the warm press box at Giants Stadium covering the Giants–Washington NFC Championship Game on a bitter cold, windy day. Allison and I wouldn't meet for another five months, so I had no idea that my future wife was at the game watching from her seat in the lower level of the stadium. She traveled by bus from Manhattan to the game after buying a scalped ticket for $300. Of course, when she told me that story on our first date, I admired her devotion but questioned her judgment.

I'm always inspired by my three amazing kids, Michelle, Emily, and Andrew, who as usual encouraged me every step on the way, and my brand-new daughter-in-law, Sophie. They all have great careers, and I'm so proud of who they are and their accomplishments. They weren't born in time to experience the '86 Giants, but trust me they heard enough about them during my research and writing process. And I can't forget my little boy Brady, my eight-year-old Cavalier King Charles spaniel, who faithfully hung by my side and took me for walks every afternoon. Yes, my kids named him after a main character in one of my books.

I appreciate my editor Ben Adams from PublicAffairs recognizing the importance of this project and sharing my vision to focus on the '86 Giants to tell the story of life after football that faces more than fifteen thousand living former players. Thanks to my agent Susan Canavan from the Waxman Literary Agency for her guidance. Thanks to Jerry Pinkus, the Giants photographer, who went through his archives from the 1986 season to come up with some unique pictures.

Of course, I really want to thank all the players and coaches from the '86 Giants who were so generous with their time and allowed themselves to be vulnerable detailing their personal and often painful stories.

Finally, I want to thank my parents, who I miss very much. My dad and I watched so many games together in our living room, and my mom always timed Sunday night dinner for halftime of the 4 p.m. games.

How lucky was I?

APPENDIX ONE:
1986 NEW YORK GIANTS ROSTER

#	Player	Pos	G	GS	Age	College
2	Raul Allegre	K	13	0	27	Texas
24	Ottis Anderson	RB	8	0	29	Miami
67	Billy Ard	OG	16	16	27	Wake Forest
58	Carl Banks	LB	16	16	24	Michigan State
89	Mark Bavaro	TE	16	15	23	Notre Dame
60	Brad Benson	OT	16	16	30	Penn State
64	Jim Burt	DT	13	13	27	Miami
53	Harry Carson	LB	16	16	32	South Carolina State
44	Maurice Carthon	RB	16	16	25	Arkansas State
25	Mark Collins	DB	15	9	22	Cal State-Fullerton
3	Joe Cooper	K	2	0	26	California
77	Eric Dorsey	DE	16	0	22	Notre Dame
28	Tom Flynn	DB	2	0	24	Pittsburgh
30	Tony Galbreath	RB	16	0	32	Missouri
61	Chris Godfrey	OG	16	16	28	Michigan
54	Andy Headen	LB	15	0	26	Clemson
48	Kenny Hill	DB	16	16	28	Yale
15	Jeff Hostetler	QB	13	0	25	West Virginia
74	Erik Howard	DT	8	2	21	Washington State
57	Byron Hunt	LB	16	0	27	Southern Methodist
88	Bobby Johnson	WR	16	12	24	Kansas
68	Damian Johnson	OT	16	0	23	Kansas State
52	Pepper Johnson	LB	16	0	22	Ohio State
59	Brian Johnston	C	4	0	23	North Carolina

Note: Pos: Position; G: Games, GS: Games started. Source: footballdb.com.

#	Player	Pos	G	GS	Age	College
51	Robbie Jones	LB	16	0	26	Alabama
43	Terry Kinard	DB	14	14	26	Clemson
5	Sean Landeta	P	16	0	24	Towson
47	Greg Lasker	DB	16	0	22	Arkansas
86	Lionel Manuel	WR	4	4	24	Pacific
70	Leonard Marshall	DL	16	16	25	Louisiana State
75	George Martin	DE	16	16	33	Oregon
80	Phil McConkey	WR	12	0	29	Navy
87	Solomon Miller	WR	16	2	21	Utah State
20	Joe Morris	RB	15	15	26	Syracuse
84	Zeke Mowatt	TE	16	5	25	Florida State
63	Karl Nelson	OT	16	16	26	Iowa State
65	Bart Oates	C	16	16	27	Brigham Young
34	Elvis Patterson	DB	15	7	26	Kansas
55	Gary Reasons	LB	16	16	24	Northwestern State
66	William Roberts	OG	16	0	24	Ohio State
81	Stacy Robinson	WR	12	10	24	North Dakota State
22	Lee Rouson	RB	14	1	24	Colorado
17	Jeff Rutledge	QB	16	0	29	Alabama
78	Jerome Sally	DT	16	1	27	Missouri
11	Phil Simms	QB	16	16	31	Morehead State
56	Lawrence Taylor	LB	16	16	27	North Carolina
9	Bob Thomas	K	1	0	34	Notre Dame
83	Vince Warren	WR	4	0	23	San Diego State
73	John Washington	DE	16	0	23	Oklahoma State
27	Herb Welch	DB	16	2	25	UCLA
23	Perry Williams	DB	16	16	25	North Carolina State

Note: Pos: Position; G: Games, GS: Games started. Source: footballdb.com.

APPENDIX TWO:
1986 NEW YORK GIANTS
SCHEDULE AND RESULTS

Week	Date	W/L	Opposing Team	Giants	Opp.
1	Mon., September 8	L	at Dallas Cowboys	28	31
2	Sun., September 14	W	San Diego Chargers	20	7
3	Sun., September 21	W	at Los Angeles Raiders	14	9
4	Sun., September 28	W	New Orleans Saints	20	17
5	Sun., October 5	W	at St. Louis Cardinals	13	6
6	Sun., October 12	W	Philadelphia Eagles	35	3
7	Sun., October 19	L	at Seattle Seahawks	12	17
8	Mon., October 27	W	Washington Redskins	27	20
9	Sun., November 2	W	Dallas Cowboys	17	14
10	Sun., November 9	W	at Philadelphia Eagles	17	14
11	Sun., November 16	W	at Minnesota Vikings	22	20
12	Sun., November 23	W	Denver Broncos	19	16
13	Mon., December 1	W	at San Francisco 49ers	21	17
14	Sun., December 7	W	at Washington Redskins	24	14
15	Sun., December 14	W	St. Louis Cardinals	27	7
16	Sat., December 20	W	Green Bay Packers	55	24

PLAYOFFS					
Game	Date	W/L	Opposing Team	Giants	Opp.
Divisional Round	Sun., January 4	W	San Francisco 49ers	49	3
NFC Championship	Sun., January 11	W	Washington Redskins	17	0
Super Bowl XXI	Sun., January 25	W	Denver Broncos	39	20

Source: ProFootballReference.com.

INDEX

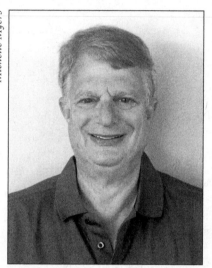

GARY MYERS is the former NFL columnist for the *New York Daily News* and *Dallas Morning News*. He is the author of six books, including the New York Times bestseller *Brady vs. Manning,* an inside look at the greatest rivalry in NFL history. Myers has been covering the NFL since 1978. He was a longtime member of the cast of HBO's *Inside the NFL* and the YES Network's *This Week in Football.* Myers is a graduate of Syracuse University's Newhouse School of Public Communications and a former adjunct professor at Syracuse. He is a voter for the Pro Football Hall of Fame.

PublicAffairs is a publishing house founded in 1997. It is a tribute to the standards, values, and flair of three persons who have served as mentors to countless reporters, writers, editors, and book people of all kinds, including me.

I. F. STONE, proprietor of *I. F. Stone's Weekly*, combined a commitment to the First Amendment with entrepreneurial zeal and reporting skill and became one of the great independent journalists in American history. At the age of eighty, Izzy published *The Trial of Socrates*, which was a national bestseller. He wrote the book after he taught himself ancient Greek.

BENJAMIN C. BRADLEE was for nearly thirty years the charismatic editorial leader of *The Washington Post*. It was Ben who gave the *Post* the range and courage to pursue such historic issues as Watergate. He supported his reporters with a tenacity that made them fearless and it is no accident that so many became authors of influential, best-selling books.

ROBERT L. BERNSTEIN, the chief executive of Random House for more than a quarter century, guided one of the nation's premier publishing houses. Bob was personally responsible for many books of political dissent and argument that challenged tyranny around the globe. He is also the founder and longtime chair of Human Rights Watch, one of the most respected human rights organizations in the world.

. . .

For fifty years, the banner of Public Affairs Press was carried by its owner Morris B. Schnapper, who published Gandhi, Nasser, Toynbee, Truman, and about 1,500 other authors. In 1983, Schnapper was described by *The Washington Post* as "a redoubtable gadfly." His legacy will endure in the books to come.

Peter Osnos, *Founder*